The Alkaline Diet Made Easy:

Reclaim Your Health, Lose Weight & Heal Naturally

Copyright Notice

Disclaimer

Claim This Now

Autoimmune Healing Transform Your Health, Reduce Inflammation, Heal the Immune System and Start Living Healthy

Do you have an overall sense of not feeling your best, but it has been going on so long that it's actually normal to you?

If you answered yes to any of these question, you may have an autoimmune disease.

Autoimmune diseases are one of the ten leading causes of death for women in all age groups and they affect nearly 25 million Americans.

In fact millions of people worldwide suffer from autoimmunity whether they know it or not.

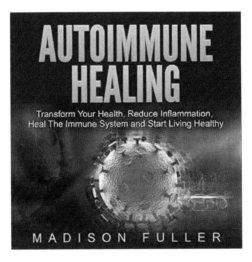

Want More?

*Sign up to get the exclusive Madison
Fuller e-newsletter, sent
out a few times a week:*

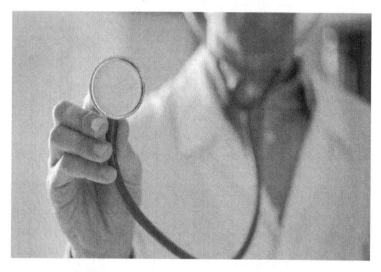

https://www.subscribepage.com/autoimmune

TABLE OF CONTENTS

INTRODUCTION

The alkaline diet keeps the body free from all the toxicity that can lead to fatal diseases. That is why the significance of the diet is more popular today than ever. Alkaline recipes are designed to bring new and innovative recipes while keeping the average pH level of the meal as basic as possible.

This guidebook comprises simple ideas and practices to start taking care of your health in the best way, adopting a lifestyle that is full of harmony and without any stress or worry. You will learn the techniques of food preparation and combination, as well as how to forge solid habits to ensure the success of the alkaline diet over time.

There are 50+ delicious, eye-catching, quick and easy to prepare recipes in this book to ensure that your taste is well taken care of and you won't get bored with your everyday meal.

What Is Alkaline Diet

Alkaline Diet is an antacid eating routine stresses soluble nourishments, for example, entire foods grown from the ground and certain entire grains, which are low in caloric thickness. Sound Alkaline Diet Foods include the perfect harmony in the middle of acidifying and alkalizing nourishments.

The body incorporates various organ frameworks that are proficient at killing and taking out abundance corrosive, yet there is a farthest point to the amount of corrosive even a sound body can adapt to successfully.

The body is equipped for keeping up a corrosive soluble parity gave that the organs are working legitimately, that a very much adjusted basic eating regimen is being devoured, and that other corrosive delivering elements, for example, tobacco use, are kept away from.

What is PH?

Generally speaking, pH is a component of our blood known as the Potential of Hydrogen.

Using the value is pH; it is possible to assess if a liquid is alkaline or acidic. In the case of human beings, we measure the acidity or alkalinity of the bodily fluids and tissues.

The importance of pH to the human body

The pH of the blood is 7.35 through 7.45, and the maintenance of this particular pH is referred to as acid-base homeostasis. This homeostasis is very important from a medical standpoint as it can be a clue toward a possible underlying medical condition, and it also has a direct impact on bodily activities, such as respiration. Acidosis, the state of having a blood pH of below 7.35, is often caused by too much carbon dioxide in the blood, and the typical response of the respiratory system is to trigger the lungs to expel this excess carbon dioxide, leading to hyperventilation. This is merely one example, albeit an important one, of the direct impact that pH can have on the human body and the importance to the human body of maintaining a safe pH.

If acidosis is left untreated, the lungs will eventually give out, leading to no respiration at all and eventual death. Indeed, the pH of the blood is so significant in terms of respiration that the medical field has a specific test, the arterial blood gas, designed to measure it. This involves obtaining a small sample of blood from a major artery in the limbs (the radial artery) with the goal of determining accurately the pH of oxygen-rich blood from the lungs (as opposed to oxygen poor blood that is heading toward the lungs in order to be replenished with oxygen). This is why the arterial blood gas, or ABG, is measured from an artery rather from a vein. Arterial blood gas samples are quickly analyzed in order to determine the best course of action for someone with a respiratory or another organ issue as these issues are often life threatening.

Again, this is merely one example of the significance of pH in the human body. The pH of extracellular fluid or ECF (the fluid outside of the body's cells, which therefore includes the blood) as carefully regulated as part of the body's normal acid-base homeostasis. This is not only because the organs of the human body have carefully evolved to detect and respond to abnormalities in the pH of the blood and other extracellular fluid in the body, but because various compounds in the body require a certain degree of acidity or alkalinity in order to function properly. A pH that is too low or too high may cause a protein or chemical in the blood to no longer function.

Proteins can become denatured (lose their shape) outside of normal physiologic pH and this can naturally lead to death. Many of you (the more dramatic among you) may think of the xenomorphic extraterrestrial from the Alien series of movies when you think of the effect of pH (specifically acid) on living things. The xenomorph alien has acid for blood and what does that acid do when it touches a surface? It burns through that surface (even metal) and would easily burn through human or other organic tissue. Now that is clearly an exaggeration of the effect that acid can have on living tissue; in reality, a pH of ECF that is only slightly below physiologic pH can be enough to denature a protein, disturb chemical processes occurring across a cell membrane, and lead to death. You do not have to be burned with an acidic compound with a pH of 2 from a xenomorphic alien in order to die because of ph. A blood or other ECF pH of the low 7's would be enough to cause death.

Maintaining a ph. balance

Do you want to know the ultimate secret to maintaining a pH balance? It's YOU. Yes, you! There are so many things you can do to achieve that, such as the following:

Test your pH level.

You can have an idea if you're acidic or not by conducting certain pH level tests. Normally if you're taking a urinalysis test, the pH level is already included in the result. However, doing this can be quite time-consuming and expensive. If you want something cheaper, you can use a pH test strip.

It is usually a kit that includes an acid-and-base-sensitive strip. You can use your urine or saliva for it, depending on the directions included in the package. The kit also includes a chart, which you can use to compare how acid or alkaline your body is. Commonly, if it's very green, your body is more alkaline; on the other hand, yellow stands for very high acidity.

You can conduct the tests at any time, though it's best if you do so during the first or two hours after you've eaten. The various metabolic processes in the body can help produce a more accurate result. If you're testing using the urine, make sure you do so with the middle flow since it's less contaminated with bacteria that may provide an inaccurate reading. If you're using your saliva, don't drink water; otherwise, the result is expected to go alkaline.

Know which body parts need to be acidic.

As we mentioned in the previous paragraphs, the goal isn't to turn the body very alkaline. That's still an imbalance, and it can cause a number of health issues. It helps you deal better pH balance therefore if you know and understand which body parts need to be acidic. For example, the stomach needs to maintain a pH level of around 2 or 3 in order for it to digest food very well. The intestine, on the other hand, can have different acidity level depending on the location in it. The duodenum, which is closer to the stomach, is acidic, but the small intestine is alkaline because of the secretion of the pancreas (see the natural balance there?). The skin, the largest organ in the body, is also acidic, since the acid gives it a natural defense against bacteria.

Drink water—lots of it.

What's the easiest way to turn your body into alkaline? Water! Water makes up the biggest portion in the body—70 percent. That's why you can live not eating for more days than not drinking. But beyond that, water is composed of two natural substances: hydrogen and oxygen. When the body has too much acidity, it actually has lesser oxygen. Moreover, lack of oxygen can lead to the overproduction of acid known as lactic acid. It happens when the body is constantly on the move but lacks the fuel because it is not receiving sufficient energy. As a result of anaerobic respiration, the body releases lactic acid, which then leads to muscle fatigue. If you have a very high level of this, even if you're not doing a lot, you can easily feel very tired. Besides, water is so much better than carbonated beverages and even coffee, which can cause dehydration. Water doesn't have any nutrients, but it also doesn't have any calorie, preservative, or anything that can cause imbalance in the body. It's completely neutral.

Eat alkaline.

We've already identified the many foods that can help turn your body alkaline. As you go along the other pages, you will read more about them. We give you a set of cheat sheets at the end of this book so you can jump start your alkaline food plan as soon as possible.

Except for a few exceptions, most fruits and vegetables are alkaline-forming, which means even if they taste sour, they are actually good for increasing the base or the alkalinity. This happens because the body's metabolic processes produce different results depending on what you're eating. In other words, too, you need to add more fruits and vegetables into your diet. A good meal should be composed of at least 80 percent alkaline-forming food and 20 percent acidic. There's no need to go raw if you're not yet ready, but take note that a lot of oils are acid-forming. Also, heating ingredients may cause the depletion of nutrients in the long run.

Learn the art of substitution.

Perhaps you may start complaining that going for alkalinity is restrictive. I understand. Everything is definitely easier said than done. But here's something great: you can do substitutions! For example, if you're raring to drink something sweet, you can add some cinnamon, cucumbers, and lemons into your water. It's even a great summer drink! You can also create a fantastic green smoothie with kale, apple, and celery. Instead of red meat, why don't you try tempeh or tofu? On its own, they don't have any taste, but they're such great substitutes to meat since they can easily acquire the flavor of the dish. Use your imagination when it comes to whipping up delicious meals made from alkaline-forming food.

Use my plan.

I've been in your position in the past, and do know it's not the easiest journey to health and wellness. I've fallen off the track a few times and have sometimes wondered if I could still do it. But I persevered, went through some trial and error, and disciplined myself. I cannot control your eating behavior or your habit. It's something that you yourself have to formulate. You need to have the will and the commitment to do this. Nevertheless, things will be a lot more convenient, easier and achievable for you when you use the easy-to-follow eating plan and cheat sheets in this book.

Reduce stress.

To achieve and maintain an optimal pH balance you should reduce stress as much as possible. Truth be told, stress forces your body to go through a period of imbalance, which, over time, can lead to acidosis or a very high level of acidity. You'll also make poorer decisions, especially when it comes to food, when you're under a lot of stress.

CHAPTER 1

In recent years, more researchers have begun looking at the alkaline diet and the stated benefits. Knowing about some of this research will help you to see why this diet became so popular so quickly.

When you eat more alkalizing vegetables and fruits, then the greater protection you will have for your muscles and bones. These foods can improve your muscle strength and decrease the chances of bone density reduction and muscular degeneration from occurring as you age. This was concluded in a study published in March of 2011 in the International Journal for Vitamin and Nutrition Research.

Preventing disease and prolonging your lifespan is a goal most of us surely have. However, you also want to stay healthy and active for every year of your life. One recent study looked at pH and its effect on your mortality and morbidity associated with various common Western diseases, such as hypertension, arthritis, low bone density, diabetes and vitamin D deficiency. This study concluded that sticking to an alkaline diet to balance pH can reduce the risk of getting these ailments and will help contribute to a longer and healthier lifespan. This study was published in October 2011 in the

Journal of Environmental Health.

One benefit not often discussed is how the alkaline diet might help to reduce chronic pain. A study was done about this topic in 2001 in the Journal of Trace Elements in Medicine and Biology. The study looked at patients who took an alkaline supplement in an attempt to alleviate their pain. A total of 82 patients took part in this study which lasted for four weeks. At the end of the trial, 76 out of the 82 patients reported that their back pain was significantly less after they took the alkaline supplements regularly.

A lot of alkaline diet research focused on its impact on cancer. One study showed that when the body has more alkaline, cancerous cell death was less likely. This study was published in October 1991 in the British Journal of Radiology. Other research has shown that cancer prevention may also be easier with this diet because of its ability to reduce inflammation.

This is certainly a lot of information to take in, but do not get overwhelmed. Now that you understand all of this, it will make it much easier to learn the intricacies of this diet. It will also aid you once you get to the final chapter and start getting ready to transition into implementing the alkaline diet as a part of your lifestyle. The next step is to dig deeper to better understand the overall effects of alkaline and acid in the body.

What Makes the Alkaline Diet Different?

The reality is that there are so many diets to choose from that we would be hard-pressed even to list them all, let alone explain them. You did not have to choose the Alkaline Diet for yourself as you might have chosen from among dozens of other diets to achieve your goals, whatever they may be. In this section, we seek to explore briefly what makes the Alkaline Diet different from other diets.

We touch on this in greater detail in the Frequently Asked Questions section at the end of the book, but essentially what makes the Alkaline Diet different from other diets is that individuals generally are embarking on this diet for reasons that are different from those that might lead them to embark on another diet. You know why you are embarking on this particular diet, and our guess is that weight or fat loss, though it may be part of the reason, is not the only reason. The Alkaline Diet falls into the category of a holistic or homeopathic diet, which means that it is part of a routine to achieve health benefits by tapping into a more natural life style. Individuals that are embarking on the Alkaline Diet often do have a desire to achieve weight loss, but this may be part of a general picture to be healthier, feel healthier, and to cleanse the body.

In reality, a diet is just that: it's a pattern of eating that dieters typically embark on for a specific reason. The Alkaline Diet is different from other diets as, with this diet, dieters are focused on the alkaline qualities of the foods they are eating rather than on the calories. Most diets involve various forms of caloric restriction, whether it is a general reduction in calories or a reduction of just fat or carbohydrates, for example. This is the means by which diets like a Low-Fat Diet, Ketogenic Diet, or Paleo Diet work to achieve fat loss, by using caloric restriction and macronutrient ratio to trigger fat loss.

The Alkaline Diet does not work this way. Although the Alkaline Diet has been shown to cause weight loss, it does not do this by specifically targeting calories. The truth is that the Alkaline Diet often does result in less caloric intake as the foods in this regimen are generally lower in fat compared to the acidic foods in many people's diets, so this is one means that weight loss can be achieved. Again, this is not the primary means by which the Alkaline Diet works. In fact, weight loss on the Alkaline Diet is often triggered homeopathically. By helping your body achieve homeostasis more easily, and by shifting away from heavily processed foods that force the body to expend energy to digest them and which also screw around with your metabolism, the Alkaline Diet makes it easier for your body to metabolize and process foods, which can reduce fat storage and improve insulin resistance.

As our body shifts to a more normal, healthier pattern of handling food (because we are eating better quality, less processed, natural foods) we tend to lose weight if we are overweight. We may also experience other unexpected effects like a fresher, healthier skin tone, improved hair texture, and the like.

This is essentially how most homeopathic regimens work. The idea is that you are replicating the manner in which your body is supposed to process foods and, in doing so, you approve the efficiency of body processes, which leads to feeling happier, healthier, and more energetic.

Reset & Reboot Your Body

The human body is one the most complex structure ever made by the universe or nature or God. And this complex structure also works efficiently and has the power to create changes in the world and create a legacy. This is the body which fights the wars, which conquers the Mt. Everest, which crosses huge oceans and islands. This is the body which invented the wheel, the electricity, the phone, the internet, and the list is endless. This body is a source of energy and ideas which have the power to create whatever the holder of the body intends. The body is a mere instrument but it is the only instrument needed to create a change in the society and the universe.

This body is made to love, to romance, to write poetry about. No wonder, the greatest hit by John Mayer "Your body is a Wonderland" speaks about candy lips, porcelain skin and bubblegum tongue. The human body is a true marvel of the nature, worth replicating but impossible to do the same.

Detoxification of your body is very necessary. Detoxification is a natural process that our body does to cleanse and remove all the unwanted materials or toxins. What we necessarily do in the process of detoxification is that we improve the natural detoxification system of the body. We just have to monitor and control the amount of toxins getting into our bodies and also to provide the nutrients needed for the body's detoxification system.

Normally, we brush our teeth, bath and shampoo our hair, use perfumes to make us smell good. Looking good does make us feel good, so is detoxification, but here is where the problem lies-people are not aware how they are abusing their body by not eating right, not monitoring what toxics they are stuffing into their bodies. And one more problem is people don't get to know when their detoxification system is not working properly.

Medically, the detoxification system is a very important system for the proper functioning of the body. In a way, our body is self-sustaining as it has the mechanisms to get rid of the toxins and wastes out of the body by itself. It produces those chemicals, enzymes, vitamins and minerals which are required to expel the unwanted toxins from the body. As the owners of our bodies, it becomes our duty to provide our body the nutrients needed to produce these chemicals to cleanse and detoxify the body.

Cleansing the body is a process. It involves a certain diet which provides the body the nutrients it needs and avoid that food material which might produce toxins in the system.

CHAPTER 2

To start the alkaline diet, prepare yourself for a lifetime of dietary changes. It is not a short-term, one-time only diet like most people associate with the term "diet". It is a long-term decision. Knowing the right foods that produce the desired healthy benefits will greatly help you succeed in making your body more alkaline.

Change how you view food

The very first step is to change the way you look at and treat food itself. Take this time to evaluate yourself. Is food merely for sustenance? Is it merely a source of calories? Or is it a source of energy and materials that the body can use to be healthy?

Food should not just be a source of energy. If this is your view, you are most likely to be not too concerned on quality. Rather, it's more on quantity. The right thinking should be on the quality of food. The alkaline diet teaches you to be more aware of the things you eat and how it ultimately affects the balance in your body. What are the ingredients in food? Does it supply the body's nutritional requirements? Does it contain potentially harmful components? What is the body's reaction to the various components of food?

Also, never think that diets are just about counting calories. What's important is that you aid your diet with exercise. Anyway, when you eat well regularly, you already get to lose around 500 calories—so there's really no need to starve yourself!

Get a list of the different types of foods and how they affect the body. A comprehensive list is available at the end of this book. Use this list as a guide on what to include in meals, what to limit and what to avoid.

Drink lots of pure, clean water

Water is vital for normal functioning of the various tissues. In fact, about 70% of the body is composed of water. It is used as a medium for various cellular processes. It is also used to dilute salts, toxins and other substances to keep them under control. Water is used as a medium for excreting wastes and toxins. It is crucial to replenish water stores in the body because it can be easily depleted through sweat, tears, urine, feces, etc.

As the human body is made up of 75% water, it comes as no surprise that a person needs to be able to sustain that amount. If a person loses water in his system, he will be dehydrated and it would be hard to live a happy and healthy life. Because of this, it's important to understand how vital water is for you and how much of it you need per day. Water also aids in weight loss. Because it has no preservatives and is not carbonated, it doesn't add any calories or carbohydrates to your body, which is essential for people who want to lose weight.

Surprisingly, water nowadays is acidic. Try to test various commercial bottled water brands and you'll see they are acidic. The usual pH range would be as acidic as pH 4 to 6. Drinking lots of water is good, but not if it's acidic. It will only add more acidity inside the body. Choose clean, pure water. If possible, get spring water, with all the natural dissolved minerals in it. Distilled water in bottles is already stripped off of all the dissolved substances that are beneficial to the body.

Sometimes, the weather gets too hot that a person may feel dehydrated. To prevent being sick or experiencing heat stroke because of extremely hot weather, it's important that a person drinks 13 to 15 cups of water per day or that he eats fruits that are loaded with fluids, too. Aside from water, a person with fever or diarrhea may also have to take oral supplements or sports drinks to replenish the loss of water in his system. You can also try fruits such as watermelons or pears—they're pretty much filled with water and that's why they are good for you.

Also, if you are fond of working out or of any activity that makes you sweat then you certainly need to drink a lot of water to make up for what you have lost. You need to add 1 to 3 more cups to your usual intake.

Aside from water, you could also drink the following:

- · Coconut Water. Coconut Water is dubbed as nature's own sports drink that has a thermogenic effect and helps make sure that the gut is strong and safe.

- · Juice. Not the processed kind, though. Try to make your own green juices (with vegetables as base), and mix and match ingredients. It's actually fun, and you'd also help yourself gain a lot of nutrients by doing so, too. Try using the following: cucumber, celery, beet, carrot, ginger, parsley, spinach, and cabbage. Then add either of the following: berries, watermelon, aloe vera, goji berry, acai berry, etc.

- · Shakes and Smoothies. Shakes and smoothies are fine, as long as you made them yourself, and they do not contain additives.

- · Tea. Herbal teas, as you may know by now, are important parts of your diet. Make sure you do not add sugar or milk, though. 3 to 5 cups per day is already good.

The lack of dissolved substances makes distilled water more acidic than regular, clean water. Instead of getting distilled water, choose filtered water. It still retains some of the valuable dissolved materials and is less acidic.

Make various meals out of cruciferous vegetables

Here's the thing: the more alkaline foods you eat, the more you lose weight. When you chew alkaline foods, it automatically means that you are already burning and digesting your food— and of course, it's only natural that you get to chew these vegetables, especially if you eat them instead of your usual snacks or fatty foods, in general. If you want to eat your snacks, you need to have the mindset of eating a whole bunch of cruciferous vegetables first—so later, you'd only eat a small amount of the snacks.

Cruciferous vegetables come from the Cruciferae Family. These are vegetables that are generally cultivated for food production. Interestingly, the name also originated from "Cruciferae", which in early Latin literally means "cross-bearing", an allusion to the shape of the flowers that seem to resemble crosses. Prime examples of cruciferous vegetables include: Brussels sprouts, bok choy, garden cress, broccoli, cabbage, and cauliflower.

These vegetables are known to be essential parts of the Negative Calorie Diet because they are high in cellulose, water, and Vitamin C, together with essential phytochemicals and nutrients that the body needs. Most cruciferous vegetables also contain glucosinulates that are said to prevent cancer, drive toxins away from the body, and could suit the taste of many—and that's why they are used in most plant-based recipes!

You see, your overall calorie intake will ultimately be reduced when you eat alkaline foods instead of high-calorie ones—and if you exercise as you do so, you'd really see substantial amount of weight loss. Once you start the diet, you'd really notice that you are losing weight. Over time, though, you might feel a lack of energy—but then you'd also realize that as your metabolism slows down, it would then work to provide you with more energy—which will then be used by your body as fuel to live!

What you should keep in mind, though, is that you have to eat at least every 2 to 3 hours—so you could sustain the energy that your body needs, and you also have to take note that you cannot eat sugar or honey—and other sugar replacements, with the exception of Stevia. It's also important not to use any artificial dressings because more often than not, they contain sugar. For dressings, you could use garlic or Dijon mustard mixed with yogurt and your choice of herbs.

Evaluate food on hand

Most of the time, there isn't any real need to throw everything that's already in the fridge or pantry and buy new kinds of food. There are no specialized food requirements for the alkaline diet. It's actually a simple type of diet, utilizing the common everyday food items. Check whatever is on hand and compare them to the list. If there are acidic foods, which is highly probable there will be, there's no need to throw them out. A great thing about the alkaline diet is that foods can be mixed to get a healthier dish.

Mix acidic foods with alkaline foods to balance out the acidity. For instance, herbs are a great way of balancing the pH of meals. Mix ginger with beef to even out the pH. Add curry spices to chicken to reduce its acid-forming effect. Not only do herbs balance the pH, these are also excellent at adding more flavor to meals. Another example of mixing foods to balance the pH is by wrapping bacon around asparagus sticks and grill or steam it. Drizzle healthy alkalizing oils over acidic foods to improve the pH. The omega-3 fats from these oils will help create a more alkaline environment in the body. Be creative. There is no need for specialized food items.

It would also help you to be on the lookout for macronutrients, also known as macros. These measure your daily intake of carbohydrates, protein, and fats. The amount that you should take might be different from everybody else's, so you do have to know exactly where you stand. For this, you have to understand that it would be important to know your measurements, starting with the size of your waist. To know the accurate size of your waist, go get a tape measure. Then, find the widest point around your belly button, and measure from there—and not from where you have placed your belt at. Then, go ahead and learn what your real weight is by weighing yourself first thing in the morning—without any clothes on.

Once you know that, you have to enter your body weight in lbs and in kilograms, and you also have to know what your body fat percentage is. If you have no idea what you body fat percentage is, you could keep the following in mind:

- · 10-14%. This is usually called the beach body look. Muscles and fat may be separated, but you may not see it in every muscle group. There might also be veins on the arms and legs.

- · 5-9%. This means that there's a lot of vascularity in the muscles—think body builders, or athletes, especially those who wrestle or play football, boxing even. The abs would also be well-defined—which means body fat is pretty low.

- · 15-19%. With these percentages, you could expect that there is less vascularity and that muscles are also not that defined anymore. You could see a great separation between them—except for the arms.

- · 20-24%. This is another common type of body fat percentage. The muscle and fat separation is almost non-existent, and the muscle groups are also not strained or vascular—making them easier on the eyes. Aim for this one.

- · 25-29%. This is already considered obese, at least, for men. This is because it's obvious how the stomach is already round, and that the waist has also increased or has widened. Neck fat may also be there, but veins and muscles may not be around.

- · 30-34%. This means that the hips are smaller than the body and waist—too much fat is visible.

This way, you would know the right portions that can help you.

Learn to listen to "hunger cues"

Pay attention to how you feel and if you know you're already hungry, go ahead and eat something, but try to scale it out. For example, ask yourself if you really are hungry in a span of 1 to 10, 10 being the highest. By questioning yourself, you'd know if you actually should eat already, but again, do not starve yourself at all.

Start slowly

To avoid getting overwhelmed with all the changes in following the alkaline diet, start slowly. Incorporate 2 to 3 alkaline meals per week. There is no need to totally change your entire week's menu just to follow this diet plan. You can start slowly as you gradually replace whatever acidic foods you have at present with more alkaline ones. Slowly add more alkaline recipes until you have at least 10 to 20 different alkaline meals per week. These meals should be tasty, so you can still enjoy the foods you want. Again, the key is to balance acidic with alkaline foods. This way, you can also curb any cravings that will come as you make the transition to a full alkaline diet.

How to Maintain an Alkaline Body

A man spends his entire life running after money and ignoring his health. The same man in his mature years is found spending the same money on the same health that he had been disregarding all his life.

 Ironic isn't it? Though there are many blessings a man does not value when in possession of health remains by and far the most neglected one among all.

People who take care of themselves not only tend to live for a longer period of time but are also more resistant to ageing.

Taking care of oneself has many aspects to it but the most important feature of a human being is his body.

With that taken well care of a person can avoid many diseases and save him of all the medication and expensive therapies that the patients go through to regain their worn-out health.

The body can be taken care of in many ways the major ones being exercise and good eating habits. The exercise being simple enough it's the eating habits that we usually lag in.

Too many desserts at a party too hard on the fats, oily food from cheap stalls that attack our blood pressure and spicy food too, give us the heart burns… all in all the guilt list goes far beyond that.

Momentarily ashamed and moved temporarily we start following fitness programs and diet charts that are soon acting as the tissues of our French fries. Restrictions forgotten all prohibitions removed we once again begin to the routine path that is destined to end up in misery. What then are we to do?

Following a diet program is easier than one might think. If you have constant motivation and a will power strong enough there is nothing that can stop you from achieving not only the ideal health conditions but also a fitness that would cut and carve your body to look smart and in shape.

There are various food that would help your body with its glow, freshness and chubbiness but the ones that provide you with strong bones, more resistant power and an energy to help improve your metabolic system should be given importance too.

All in all the cause of a lot of problems relating the body had recently been found to be the excessive acidic nature of the contents in a man's stomach. With its natural ability to produce acidic juices the body requires an intake alkaline in nature that not only neutralizes the affect of the acid present inside but also give the body spare alkali that could be used if the acid level rises overnight.

An alkaline diet is not hard to follow and consists mainly of fruits and nuts, it also prevents the patent from frequently taking in food rich in acid such as grain, citrus fruits, dairy products and the products of meat that dominates the menu of many a houses who have forgotten the importance of avoiding processed food and the increased level of acid in it.

A body that is more alkaline than acidic is a body with PH level equal to or more that 7 which is considered as neutral and neither acidic nor alkaline.

A body which acquires this state of health possesses more elastic skin and a youthful appearance. Not only in such conditions does a human have a greater mental alertness but the chances of asthma are also reduced marginally.

It provides us with more energy and reduces the chances of osteoporosis also improving the digestive system in one go. It also doesn't let yeast grow inside your body.

Needless to say people should go through this plan if not anything else for this plan does not include any side effect s and the results of the change in menu come by quickly.

 Do not follow this diet until you make sure that the level of acid inside your body is excessive. The symptoms of the body being acidic include continued exhaustion, frequent flues, irritable behavior and indigestive food followed by heart burn or acidity.

Water and alkali water can be used in these instances and the use of cucumber, seeds, carrots and bananas can reduce this level to a certain extent. Unbalanced PH level can affect our nails, give us pale dry skin and causes the hair to be dull and dead.

The acidic conditions favor osteoporosis which is commonly known as the weakening of bones and provides ideal conditions for the growth of several fatal diseases cancer being one of them.

An alkaline body on the other hand prevents the damage the acidic food causes to the teeth and mouth such as sensitivity of the teeth, the frequent bleeding and the tooth nerve pain that can be very problematic at times.

The damage not only remains to the mouth but cramping, inflammation of the eyelids, the tendency to get infected and the resistance power all in all weakens to make the body vulnerable.

An alkaline body resists these common attacks and give a man a brighter, younger and fresher look altogether. An alkaline body tends to be less depressed and less likely to have a nervous breakdown.

To get an alkaline body one must go through some steps that help a body raise its ph level slightly more than 7. A person can first of all increase the intake of all dark colored fruits and vegetable most of which are high in alkaline.

The second step of alkalizing the body is to give up on the food that is rich in acid and replace them with less acidic alternatives such as brown rice and soy beans.

A useful practice is to consume a glass of limewater prior to meals which control the amount of acid produce at that time.

Choosing fish and lamb in place of other meat products such as chicken and beef could also be a contributing factor whereas the normal oil can be replaced by olive oil. To aid the cause further vitamin C supplements could also be taken though not without consulting the doctor.

The presence of alkaline in our body is very essential though it is not an ideal practice to take large intakes of supplement and subject the body to side effects. Children should be kept away from this manner of diet and so should all pregnant and nursing women be.

Doctors are to be strictly consulted if the consumer is a heart or kidney patient an in order to prevent unfortunate mishaps.

CHAPTER 3

Benefits of the Alkaline Diet

It goes without saying that alkaline diet has numerous benefits most of which are health related. Here are some of the benefits:

More energy

Cells must function well in order for the body to produce and use energy well. Acidity interferes with proper cellular processes and reduces energy levels. By going alkaline, the cells can function better. More energy will be produced and the other cells will have more to use for their own functions. This will result to higher energy levels.

Better gum and dental health

If the body is too acidic, the oral cavity is also acidic. Acidity will cause the dental enamel to erode, which will promote the formation of dental carries, plaques and cavities. This is also among the leading causes of bad breath. The acidic environment in the mouth promotes the overgrowth of bacteria. This will cause several oral health problems such as various gum diseases. This will also increase the risk for tooth decay. Most people notice improvement in their breath and overall dental health once they go on an alkaline diet.

Better immunity

When the various cells in the body are healthy, the immune system functions better. The integrity of the cells is great. Cellular integrity protects the cells from infections. The pathogens will find it difficult to enter and cause trouble. If the pH in the body is low (acidic), the cells will find it hard to keep their structures intact. This will allow toxins and pathogens to easily enter and cause more damage. These pathogens and toxins can easily get inside the cells and alter it. This will stimulate the development of health problems. Cancer, for instance, starts off this way. This is also a major reason why some people more frequently get colds and other infections compared to those who follow the alkaline diet.

Reduction in inflammation and pain

Magnesium is an important mineral in the body. It also has a vital role in maintaining the body's pH balance. If the body becomes acidic, the cells will release their magnesium stores to help in neutralizing the acidity. The more acidic the body, the more magnesium is required to counter its effects. This may be ideal but magnesium does not only function for acid neutralizing. The body has so many other uses for magnesium. Using a lot for acid neutralizing can seriously deplete the resources for the other tissues and cellular processes to use.

One of the major tissues affected is the joint. Low magnesium in the body is one of the factors that cause joint diseases and inflammatory conditions. Also, inflammation in the other tissues in the body is also attributed to low magnesium stores.

Eating alkaline foods that are also rich in magnesium can replenish the resources and have more for the cells to use.

It strengthens the Neurons

When neurological processes are restored and protected, you get to protect yourself from Alzheimer's Disease and memory loss. Degenerative diseases could also be prevented.

This happens because alkaline foods also contain L-Theanine, an amino acid that promotes better neurological health—and not a lot of food products are able to do this.

Weight Control

This is a culmination of all the positive effects of alkalinity in the body. The cells function better, so that energy is better distributed. Fats are used properly and the body has enough energy. This will reduce cravings and hunger cues. That means reduction in the frequency of hunger cues and better appetite control. Fats and energy are also burned much better, reducing the risk of accumulating more fats that contribute to weight gain.

Preventing Stomach Upset

Thermogenesis, the term given to fat to energy conversion, is increased by at least 8 to 10 % when someone uses alkaline foods in his daily diet. This not only burns fat, but also regulates the digestive process.

Alkaline foods also reduce intestinal gas, and could also prevent certain diseases from happening, such as ulcers, ulcerative colitis, and Chron's Disease.

Slower Aging Process

The aging process is driven by the damage to cells. When cells easily degrade and repair is slow, the aging process is accelerated. If the cells are able to repair damage efficiently and at a faster rate, the aging process slows down. In an acidic environment, the cells get easily damaged and at a much faster rate. Repair is slowed in acidic pH. In an alkaline environment, cells do not get as much damage and when any injury gets repaired sooner.

Also, the aging process is accelerated due to oxidative stress. This is caused by the accumulation of free radicals and toxins that eat away at the cells. Acidic pH in the body supports oxidative stress. Alkaline pH helps in reducing the toxin load and oxidative stress. These promote younger-looking, healthier cells that give a younger appearance.

Perfect for Athletes

This is mainly because they know that if they eat too much fat, their bodies would suffer, and their hearts would grow weaker—and that's never a good thing because they live such active lives. Even superstars such as LeBron James have actually pledged allegiance to the low carb diet—so why won't you?

More so, when you adhere to these diets, it would be easy for your body to turn nutrients into ketogenic energy. When you have ketones in your system, you get to perk yourself up, and you get to have enough energy to get through the day—and help you out with whatever it is that you have to do!

Plus, when it comes to weight loss, you really cannot expect that you'd lose weigh if you keep on eating too much fats and carbohydrates. It's just not right, and won't work well with what you have in mind. Since regular exercise is said to work best with the Alkaline Diets, you can keep in mind that you could make it a part of your life—so you could be sure that the diet would really work.

Avoiding Chronic Inflammation

Chronic inflammation is the reason why so many diseases happen. These diseases include Type 2 Diabetes, Heart Problems, and Cancer. This so happens because grains are—you guessed it—inflammatory. While you may not see the effects right away, in time, you'd notice how your body would disintegrate, and how you'd feel like you're no longer in shape, and that your health is on the downlow. When you keep on eating grains, you're just fueling up the problem instead of working on ways to solve it.

Staying away from Auto-Immune Diseases

Take a look at it this way: Gliadin, also known as the worst kind of gluten, is actually responsible for affecting the pancreas, thyroids, and the entire immune system by means of releasing antibodies that aren't meant to get out yet. When these antibodies go out, auto-immune diseases come into play and one may be afflicted with diseases such as Hashimoto's Disease, type 1 diabetes, and hypothyroidism, among others.

Incidentally, research has it that Alzheimer's Disease is often triggered by high-grain diets. It releasers blockers in the brain that could break mental processes down, and therefore lead to the deterioration of the brain.

Develop a Healthy Gut

Doctors believe that the state of your gut could affect the state of your brain. After all, when you're hungry, you tend to make decisions that are not well thought out.

As you can see, your gut is in charge of a lot of things in your body—which you often fail to see in your daily life. These things include the way you utilize fat and carbohydrates; nutrient absorption; being satiated; vitamin and neurotransmitter production; inflammation; detoxification, and immunity against diseases, amongst others.

This is also because of the vagus nerve, found in the gut, which is the longest of the 12 cranial nerves. This is the main channel between your digestive system, and your nerve cells that send signals to the brain.

In short, it would be wrong for you not to take care of your gut because it would be like a way of putting your own health in danger. Why? Well, because if the given processes above does not work right, you might be afflicted with certain medical conditions, such as dementia, diabetes, allergies, cancer, ADHD, asthma, and other chronic health problems.

Not only that, the clarity of your thoughts, and the way you feel are also affected. When you don't eat what's right for you, you might be afflicted with anxiety, depression, or other problems that won't make life easy for you.

When your gut is healthy, your brain gets to make more serotonin—the hormone that keeps you happy, and keeps your sanity in check—one that not even the best anti-depressants could give out too much, and this is why you have to make sure that you start eating right.

Avoid Vitamin-D Deficiency

Even if you consume Vitamin D, it actually depletes inside the body pretty fast, and acid makes depletion even faster. More so, WGA, or Wheat Germ Agglutinin also causes bacterial growth that kills Vitamin D, and damages the gut—and could do much worse to your body in the future.

Prevention of Dehydration

Unlike coffee and soda, alkaline food makes an amazing drink because it keeps the body hydrated, and makes sure that dehydration is prevented. Alkaline food has moisture which means that it actually has water, unlike other flavored or carbonated drinks.

Feeling So Much Better

It sounds cheesy, sure, but the thing is when you adhere to this diet combination, it's like you're giving yourself the chance to feel good again.

These days, people go through a lot of things. Their lives—possibly yours, too—could turn nasty in just a second, and it would be even harder if they don't take care of their health. So, as early as now, you should consider this book a chance for you to reverse your health—for the better, of course!

The link between alkaline diet and cancer

Over time, we have heard a lot of researchers say that acidic environments help stem the growth of cancer cells. This means that if you want to prevent the growth of cancer, you should consider eating alkaline foods and looking for methods to reduce the acidity of your blood.

Alkaline foods increase the pH levels in your body, which translates to your body becoming more alkaline in nature, reducing your risk of developing cancer. Many cancer survivors preach that eating foods that are high in alkaline can help.

Is it advisable for cancer patients to change their diets?

An alkaline diet can help prevent the risk of developing cancer, but it can't be said to cure cancer. Chemotherapy and other cancer treatments are known to be more effective in alkaline environments than acidic ones. Before you alter your diet, it is advisable to discuss with your physician or dietitian. This will allow you to know if it is good for the treatment that you are undergoing or not.

Before you change your diet, whether you have cancer or not, if you take pills of any kind, it is advisable to discuss it with your physician first.

When you discuss with your dietitian, he or she can look at what your nutrition goals are, and if changes have to be made at varying treatment steps.

The dietitian looks for ways to reduce the adverse effects that may come with any changes and see if you will face any food sensitivity.

With help from your dietitian, you can find out what diet works for you.

The side effects of alkaline diet

There are a few side effects which you should be aware of which are as follows:

Could Lead To Deficiency

Don't overdo it. You could end up reducing the consumption of certain essential nutrients, vitamins & minerals which can hurt your body. For example dairy products which provide calcium to us etc. It could happen that you might have to consume supplements to offset the deficiency. I suggest that you should ask your physician when you opt for consuming the supplements.

Pregnant Ladies

Pregnant women should consult their doctors before following an alkaline diet. You may leave out certain essential nutrients required by the body while following this diet. Pregnant women should take proper advice from their doctors to get a detailed knowledge regarding the diet & supplements etc.

Allergies

Please leave out foods that you're allergic to. If you're aware of those allergic foods, just

avoid them and try the rest. If you're not aware, I suggest you should start slowly and try small quantities of the alkaline food.

Expectations

It is really important to have reasonable & judicious expectations out of the diet. You have to give it some reasonable time to work its positive magic on your body. Expecting overnight & quick results will only disappoint you & make you sad. Follow the diet for at least 30 to 40 days. If you are obese or suffer from a similar condition, then it might take a little longer for you to lose weight. But you will notice some changes positive changes within a few days like glowing skin, shiny hair, etc.

CHAPTER 4

Diseases That Can Be Prevented or Alleviated by the Alkaline Diet

Cancer

Research has it that with the help of catechins, a form of antioxidant found in Alkaline Foods, free radicals are sought and destroyed on the spot. This only means that when free radicals are destroyed, the body gets to be saved from most diseases—as well as Cancer.

A study done in McGill University shows that Alkaline Foods's antioxidants are able to shrink tumors that are mostly found in mice. Lung Cancer risk is also lessened by up to 18%, also due to Alkaline Foods.

Now, when one has already suffered from the past, relapse could be prevented with the help of alkaline foods in the sense that an increase of green alkaline foods intake prevents cancer cells from forming, mostly by destroying mitochondria—the cell that's responsible for creating cancer cells in the body. Pancreatic, colorectal, and prostate cancer are likewise prevented.

Heart Diseases

Studies show that green alkaline foods lower LDL or bad cholesterol by up to 35%. When this happens, the heart will be protected and strokes could be prevented.

More so, alkaline foods could also prevent fat build-up. Usually, people with heavier weights are those who are susceptible to heart diseases because fat is already adamant in their bloodstream. When alkaline foods are part of one's regular diet, the more it protects the body from elements that may damage the heart.

One Japanese case study has shown that 4 out of 5 men who have added alkaline foods to their diet have shown life longevity—without any heart problems!

Arthritis

Arthritis happens because of inflammation. If you've been reading this book properly, you'd know that there are actually various kinds of alkaline foods that help prevent inflammation, especially when added with other ingredients.

The thing is, compounds found in alkaline foods reverses the effects of responses that are usually associated with arthritis, diabetes, and other inflammatory problems.

The breakdown of cartilage walls is also prevented, making sure that arthritis patients are safe from further damage. You see, alkaline foods help keep a person's condition stable, instead of letting it worsen—and that's one of the best things that it can do.

Diabetes

Another amazing thing about Alkaline Foods is that it could help normalize blood sugar levels—and doing so would prevent another one of the most debilitating diseases out there—diabetes.

This happens because alkaline foods regulate the body's glucose levels—and in turn, turn said glucose to energy. Now, when this happens, one would be stronger, and would also be able to use the energy for more important things, instead of letting a disease consume the body.

Cell and Tissue Damage

As said earlier, alkaline foods are full of antioxidants that slow the process of aging down, and that also wards diseases off. Alkaline foods also repair damaged cells, and makes sure that free radicals do not get to them. More so, these antioxidants also prevent the growth of cancer cells, as well as high cholesterol levels, and also dilate blood vessels to improve energy and elasticity in the body. This also prevents clogging of the blood, and makes sure there's proper antioxidant concentration in the body.

Autoimmune Diseases

As often reiterated in this book, you can expect that with the help of alkaline foods, the aging process is slowed down—so you could still look and stay healthy even while you're growing older. Studies done have shown a lot of promise when it comes to alkaline food's effects on the immune system—which definitely is a good thing.

Remember, alkaline food is something that you could add in your daily diet. Don't try to let all the myths about it fool you—it's definitely amazing and safe!

CHAPTER 5

Alkaline vs. Acidity in the Body

The best place to start is with pH and knowing what your body does daily to keep it regulated. The state of pH in the body must be tightly regulated or else a variety of adverse health reactions can occur. The standard is 7.35 to 7.45, and this can be measured through the blood. There are slight variations in the pH of the urine and saliva, so, naturally, the body functions best when it is slightly alkaline.

What happens when the body's pH balance is disrupted? Whether something causes excess acidity or alkalinity, the body immediately goes to work to correct the pH. The kidneys and lungs are the primary regulators.

Acidosis

The body is in a state of acidosis when there is too much acid in the body fluids. This generally occurs because the lungs and kidneys are not able to keep up with getting the excess acid out of your body. This could be due to an issue with these organs or because of too much acid being produced in the body. Even a slight shift toward acidosis can produce severe health issues.

There are various kinds of acidosis, like respiratory and metabolic acidosis for example. Issues, such as consuming too much alcohol and obesity are causes of the respiratory type. When this type is present, too much CO_2 starts to build in the body. The lungs are generally good at removing it, but if something is affecting their ability to do so, it starts to accumulate. Both excess alcohol consumption and obesity can negatively impact the normal function of the lungs which can then contribute to this.

With the metabolic type, it is when the kidneys are interrupted and doesn't properly get acids from the body. There are three other forms you should know about:

- • Diabetic acidosis

This is associated with the build-up of ketones that can make the blood too acidic. This happens when blood sugar remains high for too long.

- • Lactic acidosis

This is because of an extremely high level of lactic acid. Chronic alcohol use, low blood sugar, and heart failure can also contribute.

- • Hyperchloremic acidosis

Having this means that your body is losing too much sodium bicarbonate. This is a base that promotes alkalinity when it is at the right level. Vomiting and diarrhea can cause this type.

The most common symptoms of the respiratory type include fatigue, confusion and shortness of breath. When this condition is present in the body, serious complications can occur, such as organ failure, respiratory failure, and shock. Things, like keeping your weight healthy and avoiding alcohol, can help to prevent this.

The most common symptoms of the metabolic type include fatigue, rapid breathing, and confusion. In the most severe cases, shock is possible. Increasing alkalinity is critical to prevent this type.

Alkalosis

This state occurs when the levels of carbon dioxide are too low, or bicarbonate is too high. Symptoms can include:

- Muscle twitching
- Nausea
- Hand tremors
- Lightheadedness
- Muscle spasms
- Tingling and numbness
- Vomiting Confusion

Eating a proper diet and ensuring good overall health is critical for preventing this. Not only does the alkaline diet help to keep acidity in check, but it promotes balanced alkalinity too.

Acid-Base Balance

This section will look at what the body does to keep your pH in check. The lungs are responsible for getting carbon dioxide out of the body. Carbon dioxide is a type of waste product, and it is mildly acidic. The body is constantly making it when it processes the oxygen that all of the body's cells need. It gets into the blood for excretion. The lungs pick it up and get it out of the body when you exhale. When it starts to build up, acidity occurs.

The kidneys are next. They are responsible for getting excess bases and acids out of the body. They are capable of essentially altering excretion speed in an attempt to balance the pH levels of the body. However, the kidneys do not work as quickly as the lungs when it comes to getting pH levels back on track.

The photo above provides a visual representation of where you want your pH to be once you test it. You will test it with your urine or saliva. The ideal range for both is 6.8 to 7.2. Anything below the 6.8 means that your pH level is too acidic, and it is time to make some changes. As you learned above, your body's lungs and kidneys will do some of the work. However, having the right diet is also imperative.

Why Worry About Acidity?

Acidity is the state that most people focus on because a number of maladies have been attributed to it. A body that is too acidic cannot fully heal itself. This can allow minor issues to essentially spiral out of control with time. The alkaline diet focuses on ensuring that your body remains in the proper pH balance so that should illness or injury occur, your body will use its natural healing tools to help you to recover.

When your body is too acidic and remains in this state, you are at a higher risk of being afflicted by the following:

- Hormone issues
- Weight gain
- Immune deficiency
- Free radical damage
- Stressed liver function
- Slowed elimination and digestion
- Tumor growth
- Cardiovascular weakness
- Kidney and bladder concerns
- Structural issues, such as joint troubles and weakened bones
- Low energy
- Overgrowth of fungus or yeast

The body has a number of natural mechanisms that it uses to fight off foreign invaders and promote healing. You will get the details on these just below. Just keep in mind that in order for your body to heal itself, it needs to have the right pH and the proper nutrients to fuel the processes. A largely plant-based diet provides all of these nutrients, and the alkaline diet happens to be largely plant-based. Being in a slightly alkaline state also makes it much easier for the body to fully absorb and utilize the nutrients that you are consuming. As you can see, the right diet is critical if you expect to improve your health and sustain it over the long-term.

When it comes to preventing many illnesses, your immune system is your first line of defense. It can protect you from a wide variety of infectious organisms like viruses, parasites, bacteria, and fungi. However, to function correctly, it requires specific nutrients:

- Vitamin C
- Vitamin E
- Vitamin B6
- Vitamin A
- Vitamin D
- Folate
- Selenium
- Iron
- Zinc

Your immune system has white blood cells that work to protect you. These are referred to as lymphocytes. The lymphocytes in the body will travel throughout the bloodstream and lymphatic system, while others remain in the lymphoid organs. There are many kinds of lymphocytes that fight and help to prevent you from getting sick. The 'B cells' work to produce an array of different antibodies and they release these to fight invasive foreign organisms. Then, you have the 'T cells,' which come into action to kill any cells in the body that were negatively affected by the foreign organisms.

Wounds, such as scrapes and cuts, heal in a different way. This process too requires a slightly alkaline environment and the right nutrients:

- Protein
- Vitamin A

- Vitamin C
- Zinc

All of these nutrients are easily found in the alkaline diet since they are heavily present in plant-based foods.

The wound healing process happens in stages. The first is blood clotting to prevent further bleeding from happening. Once the clot is present, it turns into a scab. It is important to leave this in place because it protects against infection.

During the next stage after scab formation, the immune system will go to work and try to inhibit an infection from setting into the wound. During this time, it is common to see some redness, swelling and tenderness. At this point, a clear liquid can be seen oozing from the scan.

Stage three is when the tissue starts to rebuild and grow. This takes an average of three weeks to complete. Granulation tissue fills the wound and any blood vessels that were damaged start being repaired by the body.

Lastly, a scar forms. This is the stage where the wound is getting to the final stage of healing and becoming stronger. If your pH is too acidic, this wound healing process can take much longer. This is because the body is not able to efficiently repair cells that are damaged in an acidic state. The negative impact on the immune system can also increase the risk of a wound being infected while it is in the healing stage.

Now you can see why getting to a slightly alkaline state has become such a major concern in recent years. A number of issues can arise when the pH of the body is out of the normal range. The alkaline diet helps to get your pH to slightly alkaline and keep it there. This can aid you in avoiding all of the scary issues that were discussed in this chapter.

CHAPTER 6

Foods That Promote Alkalinity

The primary focus of an alkaline diet is one primarily consisting of foods that have high-density nutrition. By switching to a primarily plant-based diet, you can ensure you are getting a good balance of nutrients and minerals necessary for your body to achieve a balanced pH. Here are some good choices in each of the food groups.

Fruits and Vegetables

Fruits and vegetables are one of the best foods for your body. They are low in calories, high in vitamins, minerals, and nutrients, and are packed with other beneficial compounds that improve health. Some of the most beneficial superfoods are dark, leafy green vegetables like kale and spinach. These are rich in chlorophyll, which alkalizes the blood and helps detoxify the liver. Another good source of chlorophyll is seaweed like spirulina, ALA, and chlorella, which can easily be sprinkled on top of a smoothie.

Berries are another good fruit. While some are slightly acidic, they are packed full of minerals necessary to promote health and help bring balance to your body. They are considered superfoods because of their nutritional profile. Among the healthiest are blueberries, blackberries, cranberries, strawberries, and raspberries.

As you choose fruits and vegetables each day, keep in mind that they lose some of their alkalinizing minerals when they are cooked. Uncooked fruits and vegetables, by contrast, are full of the same nutrients they had when they came from the ground. A good alternative to eating raw is juicing your produce, adding it to smoothies, or lightly steaming it so that it is not cooked all the way through.

Herbs

Herbs are a great source of vitamins and minerals. As an added benefit, you can easily sprinkle them on top of whatever you are eating for a nutritional boost. Some of the most alkaline herbs include dill, parsley, and cilantro. Fresh herbs are ideal, especially since it is easy to maintain a small herb garden in your kitchen window. However, you will get some of the nutritional benefits from dried herbs as well.

Plant Proteins

As red meat, eggs, and other protein sources typically have high levels of sulfur and can be difficult for the body to digest, plant-based proteins are a better alternative for improving alkalinity. Some good plant proteins include lima beans, navy beans, almonds, and other types of nuts and beans. You can make bean soup (with bone broth for an added benefit) or create a trail mix of dried fruit and almonds for an easy snack.

You do not have to quit eating meat altogether on the alkaline diet. However, the alkalinity of meat does not always depend on its own pH—but the way that your body digests it. This is the reason that tough red meats are harder to digest than fish. Additionally, the environment that meat is grown or raised in greatly affects its nutrient density and acidic load. Something else to keep in mind is that grass-fed meat is healthier than grain-fed meat. The same applies when considering grass-fed or grain-fed dairy products. Choosing grass-fed can reduce the acidic load on your body after eating meat.

Bone Broth

One of the most beneficial things you can consume for minerals is bone broth. Bone broth can be made from leftover bones of any animal. The bones are slow cooked in a pot of water on the stove with a little apple cider vinegar. The vinegar draws out the minerals, making the broth hearty and rich. Bone broth is something that has been used for years because of its incredible nutritional benefits and it is a great way to make sure none of your food goes to waste. If bone broth is not available, another option is supplements of bone broth collagen or collagen protein.

For people beginning the alkaline diet for the first time, it can be beneficial to eat a diet of vegetable juice and bone broth. After three days of following your diet, the pH of your body will be completely reset. You will be in perfect health to begin eating a more alkaline diet.

Root Vegetables

Rather than eating starches that harm acidity, consuming root vegetables help alkalinize your body. Slow roasting foods like leeks, onions, and sweet potatoes that are high in inulin help with the absorption of calcium and other minerals. The inulin in these vegetables is a prebiotic, which improves the health of the colon and improves the solubility of calcium.

Acidic Foods

Eat in Moderation or Not at All

People using the alkaline diet for the first time may mistakenly believe that they should eat only alkaline foods to achieve a better state of health. However, it is possible for your body to be too alkaline. Eating too many alkaline foods leads to a condition called alkalosis, which is characterized by the following symptoms:

- Lightheadedness
- Confusion
- Nausea
- Involuntary muscle spasms
- Muscle twitching or cramping
- Hand tremors
- Feelings of numbness or tingling in the arms, legs, or face
- Risk of catatonic stupor, coma, body shock, or death

Of course, these symptoms can also result from other conditions. If you are unable to do a pH test, you should speak with your healthcare provider to rule out other possible causes.

Foods that Create Acidity

While unprocessed, unhealthy foods are a major source of the pH balance in people eating a Standard American Diet, there are many other foods that create acidity when they are processed as well. Here are some of the foods that should be moderated or avoided to help you achieve an alkaline state:

- High-sodium foods- Preserved, canned, and processed foods have some of the highest content of table salt. This is usually contained in much higher levels than other minerals, which causes it to create acidity when it is consumed. Some other high-salt foods that should be avoided are conventional meats and cold cuts.

- Whole wheat and oat products- Surprisingly, even though grains are associated with healthy eating, they create acid in the body that lowers pH levels. The biggest problem is processed wheat and corn.

- Milk- Many people say that milk is rich in calcium and vitamin D, which are essential for bone health. While this may be true, milk actually creates acidity in the body that causes calcium to be leached from the bones, increasing the risk of osteoporosis. It is much better to get calcium from alkaline sources like leafy greens.

- Refined sugar- Fruit juices containing high-fructose corn syrup, refined sugar, sodas, and even artificial sweeteners like aspartame cause the urine to become extremely acidic. They must use minerals to create a buffer and safely pass through the digestive tract, which takes away from your cells, bones, organs, and tissues.

- Some other foods that cause high levels of acidity in the blood and urine include alcohol and caffeinated drinks, eggs, peanuts and walnuts, and processed bread, rice, pasta, and cereal.

CHAPTER 7

Symptoms Of Being Too Acidic

Now, often you might not realize that it causes all of this, but there are certain symptoms of a body that is too acidic, and they are important to know. This chapter will talk about the different symptoms of being too acidic, what it can cause, and even what might happen to important body systems because of it.

Immune Issues

Acidic environments are pretty much the breeding grounds for some of these pathogens. However, if you have a body that is high in hydrogen and other body fluids, it could keep the bad bacteria away. The germ is typically not always something that is the full cause, but instead, we should look at the terrain in order to view everything.

Often, there are some bad bacteria or pathogens that might stay dormant in the body that might not do anything, and there are others that come out to play, and often this comes about not because of the fact that you have a germ about, but instead it's the growing environment of this. The germ theory is very narrow, but if you start to look at the body's natural functions, you will start to see that sudden changes and different aches and pains might start to become slightly more obvious to those who are looking for a bit of another way to look at how germs come about.

Respiratory System

This is seen in some people who are struggling to breathe properly, such as in the case of bronchitis, asthma, and other such conditions. If you start to see that come about, you might want to get it checked out. The theory behind is that when you have tissues and organs that are pretty much filled to the brim with acidity, it can strangle the oxygen that is there. This means that the cells aren't handling things properly. Every single cell in the body needs new oxygen to get rid of the carbon dioxide, and it's a means to function properly. Often, if it's too acidic in an area, then you will see various wastes start to form, such as various infections and an increase of mucus. If you start to have breathing difficulties, then it's time you start looking at that as well.

Skeletal

For the skeletal system, your main symptom that can develop is arthritis. You've probably heard of this, and in essence, it's basically the inflammation of the joints. This is basically when you have stiffness, a sort of swelling, and some pain within these joints. The two forms that you might hear of are osteoarthritis and rheumatoid arthritis. Both of these do have ties to a pH imbalance and the acid deposits coming into the joints and other areas. Often, the accumulated acid is what will damage the cartilage. When you start to have cells that help lubricate become acidic, it then causes a sort of dryness and irritation that cause various joints to swell, and then there is uric acid that forms, which then start to feel like you have broken glass all over the place. Often, people start to get this going ion later in life, but if you want to reverse it, a good way to do so is through the alkaline diet.

Skin Conditions

Another sign of a pH imbalance that you might start to see this through the way your skin appears. Now some of us might have dry skin period, but let's start to look at how it protects itself against various injuries and infections. Often, the skin starts to become more inflamed because of the acid, and the skin doesn't function well against this. You might start to see sores and even lesions on the surface of the area. Even some skin eruptions such as pimples and rashes can be formed because of too acidic of a body. If you start to take care of yourself and stop creating too much of an acidic environment, it can really help to prevent the abrasions on the body.

Nervous System

The acidity of the body does create problems with the nervous system. It does so by taking energy out of it. You might hear of it being called enervation in some cases, and in general, a weakened nervous system can cause a weakened sense of physical, mental, an emotional situation within the system. Remember, acidity doesn't just affect one area, it can affect all areas as well.

Excreting

This is typically known for being the urinary system, and also can be part of when you defecate as well. The kidneys though are typically the biggest target in this, because one of the symptoms of too much acid in this area is that it can cause kidney stones to form. This is basically when there are alkaline minerals taken out from the bones and the body and then placed into your blood. These kidney stones feel awful, and they're not fun, so even your excretory system can be affected by this if you're not careful. It can also cause diarrhea as well if you're not careful, and that's never fun to deal with.

Muscular System

The muscles are actually affected by this as well. When you start to increase the acidity of the muscle cells, it can cause the metabolism to start to breakdown and mess up. This means that the muscles perform differently and not as well. Often, if you have an alkaline system, you will see better aerobic functions and you will have a better recovery in your body after you have a hard exercise. Often, it can even be seen in how you breathe, because in an acidic body, often the simplest task can be hard for them, such as walking and talking. It can be even a bit of a struggle carrying something small, but with a body that is alkaline, you'll be able to perform better, and you'll feel better too.

Reproductive System

Often, a bit of a problem that comes with an acidic environment is where the reproduction occurs. What might happen with some is that sexual dysfunction occurs, and there is a link between the condition the area is suffering from and the amount of acidity in the body. Often, one sees through decreased lack of arousal, or even enjoyment of sex for some women, and it can decrease the fertility of both parties, and cause one to miscarry. Your reproductive health is important, and it is imperative to remember that it's also a part of you, so you should make sure it's kept maintained as well.

These are but few of a symptom of an acidic body, and it is imperative to know that there are many more that can come about if you're not careful, and you should know them before you continue, because they can adversely affect you if you're not careful.

CHAPTER 8

Water

Blood, muscles, voice, as well as human brain, all of this major body parts contain water. You will need water to maintain body's temperature also to provide you with the method for vitamins and minerals to go to the organs and flesh.

It also helps transfer fresh air to your cells, eliminates waste, as well as shields your joints as well as internal organs. Consuming too little water contributes to lack of fluids. Signs and symptoms of gentle dehydration include thirst, aches and pains throughout muscles and joints, low back pain, headaches and bowel irregularity.

A solid odor on your urine, plus yellow-colored as well as silpada coloration, may indicate that you are not getting sufficient drinking water. Be aware that riboflavin, a B – supplement, will make your own urine vivid discolored whenever you take dietary supplements which contain huge amounts associated with riboflavin. Selected drugs can change the color involving pee as well.

An individual gets rid of normal water by means of urinating, respiratory, by excessive sweating, so you shed more normal water if you are active than if you are exercise-free. Diuretics, like caffeinated drinks pills, selected prescription drugs and also booze could raise the volume of drinking water your system loses. Misplaced body fluids have to be replaced by the particular liquids in the meals you take in as well as the refreshments an individual drink.

How much water must you drink? No less than 20 % from the water you may need comes from your diet. The others come from the beverages you consume. Several specialists believe you are able to estimation the amount of normal water you will need by taking weight in lbs and separating the time in two. Which gives the particular number of oz you might want to consume on a daily basis.

For example, in case you ponder A hundred and sixty pounds, you might like to consume at least 80 ounces of water or other liquids daily. Additional circumstances contain quantity of exercise and also the local weather what your location is situated. Our water car loan calculator may help you figure out how much water you'll want to beverage on a daily basis.

Drinking water has become the most suitable option with regard to rehydration because it is inexpensive and possesses no energy or perhaps included ingredients. Touch as well as canned ended up being is often fluoridated, to assist reduce tooth decay. Sweetened carbonated drinks as well as carbonated drinks get added sweets that contribute extra calories from fat but no added nutrients and vitamins.

Sporting activities products incorporate mineral deposits that can help keep your water in balance; however look out for included sugar as well as calorie consumption that you could not want.

Vegetable and fruit juices is usually a good option simply because they have minerals and vitamins your body needs (go through labeling, however — plant fruit drinks may be loaded with sea salt). Caffeinated liquids such as tea and coffee count number too, yet too much caffeine can make you feel nervous.

The most basic of functions within the body are entirely reliant on water. Without a sufficient supply, the blood would be unable to carry vital nutrients to the organs. Also, water is a key component in the body's ability to process waste. Thirst is a serious warning sign from the brain, which indicates that fluid is required urgently. The brain communicates with the kidneys via the Posterior Pituitary gland – it will send signals to the kidneys about how much urine should be excreted and how much is to be stored in reserve.

How much water we should drink on a daily basis has been the cause of much debate, but the official recommendation from the Department of Health is 1.2 liters per day. There has been a figure banded about, that we should consume 2.5 liters per day, but this is a confused figure, as it relates to total fluid loss per day and our total replacement requirements.

It does not follow that we should take on board the full replacement requirement in the form of drinking, as approximately 1 liter of fluid is recovered from food and a further 0.3 liters from chemical reactions. This is where the 1.2 liters per day figure comes from. To put this into context, that is 8 glasses of water, assuming that each glass holds 150ml.

The health benefits of drinking water are more far reaching than is often stated. Muscle fatigue can result from an inadequate water intake, as muscles shrivel due to an imbalance of fluid and electrolytes. There is also evidence to suggest that healthy skin can be promoted by staying properly hydrated. Your kidneys will benefit from a good supply of water, as it minimizes the amount of work they are forced to do in order to process waste. A plentiful supply of water also results in the easy flow of waste through the system, as the kidneys are not forced to withhold fluid from the urine.

Further claims abound regarding the advantages of proper hydration for the body. Dehydration has been linked to heartburn, arthritis, back pain, angina, migraines, colitis, asthma and hypertension, to name but a few. The reality is that the human body is a water-based machine. Water is the lubrication and the fuel and without an intake which compensates for the natural losses experienced day to day, the machine cannot function successfully and will eventually break down.

Alkaline Water

Alkaline drinking water contains vital magnesium and calcium, salt and also blood potassium that are nutrients inside a type which can be quickly digested by the entire body. Ion technology alterations the molecular group of water to merely 5 or 6 elements every chaos for straightforward gain access to with the system tissues.

This specific drinking water ph aids our bodies to replenish with water more rapidly and assisting regulation of body temperature pertaining to much better wellness.

In a few places that there exists insufficient calcium supplements in the water, you can add calcium supplements for the h2o ionizer and it will develop calcium supplements towards the ionized normal water to the human body's requires

The actual power billed water ph with the drinking water ionizer rearranges these types of balanced vitamins for simple compression by simply the body, which may be called electrolysis method. Ionized drinking water will help eliminate harmful poisons, raising our own degree of energy, helps our alkaline/acidic stability, moisturizing tissue, resulting in a physique abundant... along with additional electricity.

The feeling of exhaustion and feeling unsettled are among the symptoms of too much acidity in the system. Ingesting more ionized water may help this kind of situations. Once we consume alkaline water we are ingesting a robust and also all-natural anti-oxidant which renews one's body.

Ingesting the best pH water helps you to bring nutrition, combating viruses and a bacterium breach and in addition removes waste.

1. Alkaline normal water is made up of vital calcium mineral, magnesium mineral, sea salt, along with blood potassium minerals within a form which can be easily gotten from the body.

Cancer malignancy does not prosper in an oxygen rich and alkaline atmosphere.

Alkaline h2o offers a balanced ph balance that encourages health.

2. Ionized alkaline-water is made up of smaller compound groupings that assist one's body deal with far more normal water also to stay hydrated system far better.

3. Using alkaline h2o in order to reconstitute your juices coming from target will lead to a new nicer flavor; precisely the same pertaining to coffee and green teas.

Normal structure and also color is actually maintained within fruit and vegetables cooked throughout alkaline water. Grain will likely be loftier after staying boiled inside alkaline-water.

Alkaline normal water aids in weight loss, along with reduces food cravings whenever going on a diet. Ingest at the very least 8-10 ounces of water each day.

CHAPTER 9:

Can this Really Work Long Term?

Many people start to see how this makes for balanced eating and proper nutrition. At first they may think that eating in this way is difficult, but it becomes a bit easier as you move along. For many this isn't a huge chore, but rather a way of relearning what it means to eat healthy and balanced by incorporating the right foods.

After the initial time period and adjustment has passed, how can you keep the momentum of the Alkaline Diet going? Is this like every other diet or eating plan that you have tried which leaves you feeling disappointed in the long term?

Here's what you need to remember about the Alkaline Diet. It is based on solid health principles. This is a diet that was created to help those who needed to achieve better pH balance within their systems. This is not a diet about weight loss specifically, but rather working towards better health. That means that you don't have to worry about the longevity of it or the way that you can keep at it because it is a lifestyle.

You CAN do this in the long term, and if you fall off track you can easily get back on track by readjusting the amount of alkaline foods, you eat in comparison to the acidic foods. That's where the Alkaline Diet is different from so many other trends and diets out there, and why it can sustain you in the long term. There are no phases or redo's just a matter of balance.

Your Mindset Needs to Change

I am a big believer in the fact that even a well-balanced, nutritious eating plan will fall apart eventually if you do not take the time to change your mind set about eating in the first place.

The Alkaline Diet can and will help you in the long run, but only if you use it to the best of its capacity. If you view this like any other short-term diet and try to approach it with the same tired mindset, then you will fail at it and it will fail you. If you can really start to look at the Alkaline Diet as a balanced view of nutrition that will help you to give your body what it needs, then the magic will start happening. Here are a few things to consider which will help your view and approach to eating using the fundamentals of the Alkaline Diet:

- Change your mind set about the way that you eat overall. This is not a diet in the traditional sense because it is based on good health principles. So, stop looking at this as a method of deprivation or a way in which you are convinced that you will feel hungry or defeated. Try to put aside whatever happened in the past and let the focus now be on what it means to eat well and feel your best.

This is about achieving proper health through the right foods, and if you can change your mind-set at the start then you will achieve better results. This isn't just a short-term view that will only support you for a set period of time. This is instead a much longer-term view of eating the right way that will get you healthier, give you balance, and protect you now and in the future. The Alkaline Diet is totally different from anything else that you have ever done!

- If you fall off track or feel imbalanced, then just get back to basics. This isn't the type of diet where you beat yourself up if you ate the wrong foods. It's not like that as it's not about calorie counting, or writing down everything you ate, or avoiding all food groups but one. This is a balanced view of eating and nutrition in every sense.

So, when you start to see that the true balance is achieved by focusing on these foods, then it all comes together. You feel the power when you eat these foods and you may already feel a sort of internal balance because they are nutritious, whole, and good for you. If you fall off track, have a bad day, or just feel not quite yourself, then just get back to the basics and fundamentals of the Alkaline Diet. It's really that easy! No more beating yourself up or feeling bad about things, because this is very much about eating right for the right reasons and not a short-term view anymore.

- Learn to incorporate the right mix of alkaline and acidic based foods regularly. You see now what make for some of the most acidifying foods and what make for some of the most alkaline based foods. Now it's up to you to find your perfect mix, and that may even change from time to time which is perfectly okay! It's up to you to figure out how to achieve true balance and it may take a bit of trial and error as mentioned.

Good foods can mix well and make for eating right throughout the day. It may change up over time or you may need to incorporate variety to keep it interesting. You get to experiment a bit and see which will work to your advantage and what will help you to ultimately feel your best. Food has great power, and you will see that when you use the Alkaline Diet as your basis for an overall lifestyle!

- Retrain yourself to eat the right foods and it will just be your norm. It may mean that you have to forget about what you thought you knew about balanced and proper nutrition. It may mean that you have to abandon what you thought you knew and understood a diet to be. This is where you move forward with the right attitude towards food and really allow balanced nutrition to give you so much more than you ever imagined.

- This is never about deprivation but rather eating in the right way. Again, you may have to retrain yourself a bit here. Forget about calorie counting or deprivation that left you feeling hungry and bitter. You DO get to eat, and as a matter of fact focusing on the right foods and eating them regularly give you everything that you need. You may very well lose weight and you will keep it off using the Alkaline Diet because it's so healthy and sound in its basis. You aren't constantly focused on weight loss, and that may also be what helps you to achieve results. Rather than pushing to deprive yourself to lose weight, you're actually eating healthy foods and enjoying eating.

You may even stop yourself to be sure that this is really accurate or real because it feels so good to actually eat and lose weight! This is a much better eating plan and the Alkaline Diet isn't something that will consume your thoughts in an unhealthy way, but rather just acts as a basis for better eating overall. Balance in your pH levels, balance in your overall eating to help protect your health, and balance to likely help you to lose weight in the right way—but it never becomes about that or monopolizes your thoughts and perhaps that's precisely why it works so very well!

CHAPTER 10:

Alkaline Shopping

Another thing that you have to understand about the Alkaline Diet is that it is essential for you to choose proper portions. When you portion your food, it becomes easier for you to make sense of what you're eating—and because of that, you can get more of the nutrients that you need, too.

Start with meat…and all kinds of protein

So, what should make up your portions, then? First, you can start with Protein, which definitely includes turkey or chicken breasts, salmon, tuna, halibut, pork loin or pork chops, non-fat mozzarella cheese, tofu, beans, lean beef, veal, soy milk, yogurt, nuts and seeds, eggs, and egg whites.

Protein is one of the body's essential nutrients because it is very beneficial. It can repair and replace tissues, hair, blood, nails and even muscles and a person need to sustain the amount of protein in his system so that he would not easily be susceptible to diseases. For athletes, protein is important because it builds muscles instead of fat and keeps them sturdy and on their feet. Body-builders rely on Protein a lot, too. Protein is also considered as the building blocks of tissue, which means that it can also be considered as one of life's building blocks. Without it, a person will feel unhealthy and would not be able to function well.

The recommended amount of Protein always depends on your age, sex, weight and level of activity. Around 50 to 175 grams per day is generally good. This also means that you can eat at least 5 to 6 ounces of protein-rich food each day. Men also need more Protein than women. If a woman eats 6 ounces of Protein each day, a man has to eat 7 to 8. Adults also need more Protein than children and so do bodybuilders. A bodybuilder has to eat 6 to 9 grams of protein per every pound of his weight. Other active adults have to eat 4 to 5 grams of protein each day, too.

Lots of vegetables

Veggies should make up at least ¾ of your plate. Most vegetables have low acid content. Males need around 2 to 3 cups of vegetables daily while women need 2 to 2 ½ cups. The same level goes for fruits. However, the amount may change depending on the kind of activity you do, your gender and also your age. Take note that again, men need more vegetables than women and that if they are extremely active or if they do 60 or more minutes of physical activity daily, they would need 4 to 5 cups of vegetables and around 3 to 4 cups of fruits. Kids need around 1 to 3 cups of vegetables and 2 to 3 cups of fruits daily.

Vegetables help reduce the risk of heart diseases such as heart attacks and stroke and can also protect the body against certain types of cancer. Vitamin C aids against inflammation and helps wounds heal fast. Plus, it also protects the body against several types of infections. Vegetables are also great sources of essential nutrients such as Vitamin C, Vitamin A, Folate and Dietary Fiber. Fiber not only aids in weight loss but also cleans the systems of the body and rids it of toxins. Aside from that, it's also important in regulating bowel movement. When this happens, it will be easy for you to digest food and be able to get the nutrients you need from the foods you eat. Fiber heightens the body's metabolic levels, too.

As some vegetables are high in potassium, it means that they can lower your blood pressure, decrease the level of bone loss and can also help in lowering blood pressure, as well. Some vegetables that are rich in potassium include potatoes, sweet potatoes, lima beans, beet greens, lentils, soy beans, tomatoes, tomato products and kidney beans, as well. Vegetables are rich in fiber so they can prevent obesity and Type II Diabetes and can definitely aid in making you lose weight fast.

Vegetables also keep the skin healthy and radiant, and vegetables that are rich in folate are great for pregnant and lactating women. These vegetables give them a chance to produce healthier kinds of milk. Aside from this, Folate also provides the body with healthy red blood cells which means that you will not be easily susceptible to diseases and that you can absorb other nutrients easily. Folate also protects the body against certain diseases such as spina bifida, tube defects and acephaly that are easily gotten when the baby is still inside the mother's womb. As you can see, eating vegetables can help protect the baby and make sure that he gets out well and healthy.

To make portion control easier, you can make use of the following vegetables:

- Lettuce. Aside from extremely low amount of acid, what you can expect about lettuce is that no matter how much you eat of it, it still won't make you gain a lot of weight. Lettuce that contain the most nutrients are red leaf, purple, or dark green.

- Brussels Sprouts. What's great about Brussels sprouts is that they're loaded with fiber and phytonutrients that make you lose weight and that prevent cancer. Sure, you may not like them at first, but when cooked right, they actually taste amazing.

- Beets. What's amazing about beets is that although they are sweet, they actually do not contain sugar and they are also filled with fiber, antioxidants, potassium, folate, and iron!

- Mushrooms. Mushrooms are not just the favorite pizza toppings of some, they're also quite amazing because they could boost and protect the immune system as they contain fiber, B Vitamins, potassium, and loads of antioxidants! The best variants include Portobello, Shitake, and White, amongst others.

- Turnips. Turnips promise low glycemic index, which means you'll also be protected from diabetes, and is also one of the best sources of Vitamin C.

- Spinach. Another miraculous vegetable, spinach is quite flavorful. It contains Vitamin K, Folic Acid, iron, beta-carotene, and phytonutrients that help you lose weight and protect you against loads of diseases. It also prevents macular degeneration.

- Zucchini. Another favorite, zucchini is sometimes known as the "miracle squash" because it allows you to feel satiated—without filling you up with calories. It's also filled with Vitamin A!

- Garlic. Garlic is amazing because it strengthens the immune system and helps fight colds, together with most urinary infections. It has lots of antimicrobial and antiviral properties!

- Kale. One of those vegetables that are part of many diet regimens these days, Kale is a great superfood that prevents breast cancer and is also filled with lots of phytonutrients. Aside from that, it's also one of the best sources of manganese, folic acid, and most vitamins, as well.

- Carrots. They are so low in cholesterol and fat, which makes them a perfect part of this diet. They're also rich in beta-carotene and Vitamin A—essential nutrients that the body needs.

- Celery. What's great about celery is that it's filled with cellulose and it's considered a high-volume food—which means that even if you eat a lot, you won't get fat. It's perfect for those who are trying to have healthy pregnancies, and is also filled with folate, vitamin C, and vitamin A, among others.

- Fennel. This prevents winter coughs, boosts your immune system, and is filled with lots of vitamins and minerals, as well.

- Radishes. They aid in digestion because they contain lots of sulfur compounds, antioxidants, and folic acid, and has twice the amount of calcium that leafy vegetables have.

- Pumpkins. Pumpkins have many antioxidants, beta-carotene, and essential vitamins. It's also so easy to add to a lot of dishes, so it's a great part of any diet! It lowers blood pressure, as well.

Add some carbohydrates

Next, you also have to realize that carbohydrates are not actually that bad. In fact, you need a good amount of them in any healthy, balanced diet. Carbohydrates are important to your body when taken in the right amount. Carbohydrates are essential because they boost your mood and increase the amounts of "happy hormones" in your body; they keep the memory sharp; they are good for your heart and have the right amount of soluble fiber that you need. Eating 5 to 10 grams of carbohydrates daily can lessen the amount of cholesterol in your system by at least 5 percent, and; they help control the amount of fat in your body, making sure that fat gets turned into glucose—which your body could then use as "energy" or fuel to live.

For this, you can try quinoa, whole wheat pizza, barley, bulgur, or popcorn. Basically, the mount of carbohydrates that you need depends on your lifestyle. For example, people who are lean and who regularly work out need just 100 to 150 grams of carbohydrates per day. This means that they can eat all the vegetables they want together with some fruits and healthy starches such as sweet potatoes, oats and rice.

If someone wants to lose weight but still cannot give up carbohydrates, he is allowed to eat 50 to 100 grams of carbohydrates per day. This means that he has to eat plenty of vegetables, around 2 to 3 pieces of fruits and a minimal amount of starchy carbohydrates each day.

And, try some good fats

Unlike what you're usually told, fats aren't all that bad. The right kinds of fats are very good for you and necessary for a healthy diet. Good fats provide you with energy and also help your body absorb nutrients easily plus they can also control or stabilize the body's cholesterol levels so you can live a healthy and well-balanced life. You can always start with mono-unsaturated fats, or those that are found mostly in oils and certain types of food. They decrease the risk of heart diseases and also control an insulin and blood sugar level which protects you from diabetes. They also help you feel full and satiated, so small amounts of monounsaturated fats, when added to your food, can help you feel full longer.

Then, you also can eat some poly-unsaturated fats, or fats found in oils and plant-based foods that can control cholesterol levels and protect you against heart diseases and certain types of cancer.

And of course, you shouldn't forget about Omega-3 Fatty Acids, which are found in tuna and most seafoods and are good because they keep the heart healthy and can reduce the risk of coronary heart disease, artery problems and irregular heartbeats. These fats also aid in weight loss.

Fat intake depends on your age, gender and lifestyle. Generally, adults and less active women should take 1,600-2,000 calories each day while teenagers and very active women and active men should take 2,500 calories or less each day. Doctors also recommend a 2,000 to 2,500 calorie diet or 44 to 78 grams of fat per day for everyone as a total of all kinds of healthy fats.

If you're wondering where you could get healthy fats, here is a list of foods that are rich in healthy fats:

- Seeds. Seeds lower the amount of cholesterol in your body. Sunflower and Pumpkin Seeds are the best that you could try.

- Peanut Butter. This beloved sandwich spread is actually healthy for you because it is made up of mono-unsaturated fats. Choose finely ground ones instead of chunky/crispy ones with parts of nuts still in them. Choose natural peanut butter that hasn't been loaded with extra sugars. Now, you know that the classic Peanut Butter Sandwich can actually be good for you!

- Omega 3 Fortified Foods. Check labels of different food products and if you see that they are loaded with Omega 3, go for them. Oatmeal is one good example of this.

- Olive Oil. Use olive oil for cooking and you will be able to serve something healthy and good for the heart.

- Nuts. Nuts are also healthy sources of fats and what's great is that fats from nuts are good for the heart. Walnuts, Pecans and Hazelnuts provide you with ample amounts of nutrients. Make sure though that you don't eat them during every meal because it would be bad for your cholesterol levels. 1 ounce per meal per day would already be good. An ounce means around 35 peanuts, 24 almonds and 15 pecan halves. 18 cashews would also be good.

- Kale, Spinach and Brussels sprouts. These vegetables are good sources of omega 3 fatty acids that keep the heart healthy and can protect you against various diseases. 2 to 3 cups of these greens each day would be beneficial for you so don't forget to add them to your shopping list.

- Ground Flaxseed. This contains enough soluble fiber that can rid your body of toxins and that will certainly protect you against various diseases. It's also the reason why flaxseed is all the rage these days when it comes to diet regimens. Use flaxseed for cereals or salads and you'll be alright.

- Fish. As mentioned earlier, omega 3 fatty acids are examples of healthy fats and you can get those from fish such as sardines, trout, tuna, herring, mackerel and salmon. Aside from being full of healthy fats, they also aid in keeping your brain sharp and smart. 2 servings of fatty fish each week is essential.

- Eggs. Eggs are not only a good source of fat, it's a good source of protein, too. An egg per day would definitely keep the doctor away.

- Beans. Kidney Beans, Navy Beans, Soybeans and Lentils boost your mood and strengthen the body, too.

- Avocado. What's good about avocado is that you can make different dishes and dips out of it. Make a guacamole, salsa or add it in your omelets or sandwiches and you'll certainly enjoy it. It prevents osteoarthritis and is definitely good for the heart, too. A medium avocado per serving can be good for you.

Compute carb and protein intake

When you make use of proper portions, it'll be easier for you to follow the alkaline diet. You also should compute your carbohydrate and protein intake, and make sure that it falls under 1.2 grams per meal or around 30 grams each day. For this, compute the following:

1. Daily Carb Intake (grams)
2. Daily Protein Ratio (grams/lb.)

CHAPTER 11:

Secrets to Rebalance Your pH

Now that you have an understanding of the basic of the Alkaline Diet and also have an idea of what foods are the mainstay of your diet, you are ready to tackle your diet head-on. You will do that by learning the 21 secrets that are the keys to success on the Alkaline Diet. These secrets will not only aid you in better understanding the diet but reiterate the main concepts that are essential to entering your diet like Clark Kent and leaving it like Superman. It really isn't that difficult.

Secret 1: Understanding what pH is and how it works is the key to creating a normal balance in the human body and encouraging overall health. The human body seeks to maintain a certain homeostasis and specific foods that we eat can either encourage the body's natural homeostasis or derail it.

The key to achieving success on the Alkaline Diet is having an understanding of what pH is and why it is important to your health. Sure, most of us would have learned about pH in school, but that was a long time ago for many of you and one of the goals of this book is to take what you know (and maybe what you don't) and help you to redirect that information towards a healthy, happier lifestyle.

Though you do not need to measure pH of urine or other bodily fluids to achieve success on this diet, you do need to have a basic understanding of what's in foods and why it's important.

Fortunately for you, we have done most of that work for you by distilling all of that information into the two charts that you read in the previous chapter.

Secret 2: The normal pH of the human body lies between 7.35 and 7.45. A blood pH below 7.35 is described as acidotic while a blood pH above 7.45 is described as alkaline or basic.

This is not a science book and you do not have to memorize any calculations in order to be successful on the Alkaline Diet. What is it important to know, however, is that there is something called physiologic pH, and that is the natural pH that the body seeks to maintain in the blood and other extracellular fluids in order for it to engage in its normal bodily processes and achieve homeostasis.

The pH will vary depending on the type of extracellular fluid, but the normal pH for the blood is about 7.4. Remember, the body needs to maintain this pH in order for proteins and other compounds in the blood to maintain their normal shape; this pH is also important for cells in the blood and lining the blood to engage in their normal metabolic and other processes. The body actually has to expend energy to maintain this pH as this pH is necessary for life to continue.

Secret 3: Even the ancients understood the importance of consuming foods that contained a certain balance between the specific qualities of the food. The Alkaline Diet is based on the same idea.

Although the Alkaline Diet of today is based on science that was not well understood until the beginning of the early 20th century, the underlying concepts of this diet date back thousands of years. Even the ancients under the ideas of "humors" or physical qualities of the blood and body that could either cause illness or prevent it. Essentially, scientists and thinkers of the past were talking about pH and other chemical qualities of the blood and body that we did not begin to understand until the 20th century. These ancient minds were able to treat illnesses that even today we have difficulty fully treating or even understanding with solely well-thought out diet regimens. They were perceptive in ways that we can hardly imagine, and people in the past were able to live long, healthy lives on natural alkaline food sources like olive oil, fruits, vegetables, grains, and grasses.

Secret 4: The Alkaline Diet of today is based on the magical ratio of 80% alkaline ash foods and 20% acidic foods.

The Alkaline Diet of today, that we advocate for in this book, consists of partaking of a diet that is made up of 80% alkaline ash foods and 20% acid ash foods. Though some people choose to partake of a diet that is made up exclusively of alkaline ash foods, this is not necessary on this diet. Therefore, you will be able to partake of some meat, fish, or eggs (and other acidic spectrum foods) if you really want to! What's great about the alkaline ash diet, and contrary to what some people might think, is that there are many delicious, exciting foods that you can partake of in this diet.

It's not your grandmother's cod liver oil and prunes (both of which are acidic, by the way), this is a diet that you can easily convert into delicious meals every day. This is especially easy in this day and age where foods and food products from around the world are more readily available than they have ever been before. Before we dive into the next secret on the list, let's spend a moment to talk about some of these delicious foods. We have made a list of ten foods that you can incorporate into almost any meal to maintain the alkalinity of that meal.

Wheatgrass. It is simple and easy to incorporate a shot of wheatgrass into any meal, or even to have a shot at different times of the day. Wheatgrass is easily obtained at grocery stores and health food stores and it only takes a few shots here and there to obtain the varied health benefits associated with this awesome, easy alkaline food.

Tofu. Tofu is not only healthy and affordable, it can be used as an ingredient in a wide variety of foods. Made from soybeans, tofu is more readily available than ever before. You can fry eat, eat it plain, use it to make tofu burgers. The possibilities really are endless with tofu, a miracle food and a staple of the Alkaline Diet for many people.

Almonds. The great thing about almonds and nuts is that they are a dry food that it is easy to transport and snack on. And you don't have to snack on them, they can be an intrinsic part of a meal, like a salad, a vegetable dish, the list goes on. Not only that, almond milk is also derived from almonds and almond milk is a favorite for people who are either lactose intolerant or wish to keep things alkaline by staying away from animal milks (though goat's milk is considered an alkaline ash food). Many recipes these days incorporate almond milk so if you are really committed to this diet, almonds and almond milk are an ingredient that you should make great use of.

Grapefruit. Grapefruit is not only delicious, but it is easily obtainable and healthy. There was a time when people loved to snake on fruits like grapefruit, and though it may seem like those days are far in the past they do not have to be. Incorporating grapefruit into your 80% alkaline ash foods for the day will help you to easily meet your daily requirements.

Sesame Seeds. Sesame seeds are an easy alkaline ash food that can be incorporated into any food. They taste great, their easy to obtain, and their cheap. Consider having sesame seeds in your kitchen as part of your new Alkaline Diet regimen.

Tomatoes. Tomatoes are an alkaline food that many of you probably already manage to incorporate into your meals. They can easily be added to a salad or tofu burger; they can even be eaten as a snack.

Coconut. Coconuts are widely considered to be a superfood, not only because they are so healthy, they are also delicious and can be utilized in a variety of different ways, allowing them to be incorporated into many meals and recipes. Coconuts can certainly be eaten in their natural form, but they can also be consumed in the form of coconut juice, coconut oil, coconut milk and the like.

Coconuts are truly a miracle food and we recommend the coconut as a staple of your Alkaline Diet.

Avocados. Avocados are another so-called superfood and these should also be incorporated into your Alkaline Diet. They can be incorporated into many dishes and meals or they can be eaten alone. When you embark on the Alkaline Diet, you begin to realize how fulfilling it is to engage in a diet that's just as delicious and filling as a modern diet, but without all the chips and soda. You can go to sleep at night knowing that you ate heartily and well. And all it took was an avocado…

Pumpkins. Sure there are lots of things that you can do with a pumpkin, and one of the best is eating one. It does not have to be Halloween for you to enjoy the company of a pumpkin. Put some on your salad or include it with a great vegetable dish. Incorporate a pumpkin into your life today.

Watercress. All right, watercress sprouts are one of those things that you always hear about, but never manage to incorporate into your diet, but you should. They can easily be incorporated into a variety of meals. They are also low in calories and confer some great nutritional benefits. Make friends with the watercress today!

Secret 5: An Alkaline Diet can be used to treat conditions associated with acidosis of the blood or urine, including kidney stones, urinary tract infections, and osteoporosis.

This is a poorly-kept secret. Many of you embarking on the Alkaline Diet are doing so because you may be knee deep in a particular health problem and you have heard that the Alkaline Diet can help you remedy that problem. As we have reiterated many times in various locations in this book, many health problems are directly related to consuming diets that are heavy in acid ash foods. Not only that, but many detrimental states in the body cause the blood to become shifted towards acidosis, causing the body to have to work overtime to maintain a homeostasis that is not only natural, but essential for life. In reality, you do not have to be suffering from any ailment to derive benefit from the Alkaline Diet. Many people choose to partake of this diet because they want to prevent illness or medical conditions that develop later in life like osteoporosis.

Secret 6: The human body goes to great lengths to maintain homeostasis, as certain conditions (which we can summarize as homeostasis) are essential for the body to function normally.

This is another concept that is important to reiterate because it is not only an important part of the Alkaline Diet, but it is also a secret that even people in the medical community do not understand. Though the Alkaline Diet may be unique compared to other diets, it also shares some commonalities with them. Many modern diets of day work by understanding how the body works normally. For example, the Intermittent Fasting diet works by tapping into how the human body normally processes food after centuries of evolution. The human body has evolved to expect periods of fasting (when one is not eating) punctuated by periods of eating. When you are not eating, the body burns fat from its own fat stores to meet its caloric requirement. This is an example of how a diet can tap into how the body functions normally. Well, the Alkaline Diet isn't much different.

The Alkaline Diet taps into your body's own desire to maintain homeostasis by helping your body get there. Because you are assisting your body in this process, your body does not have to deal with the confusion of all of these acid ash foods flooding the bloodstream when you are already acidotic to begin with; now your body not only has to digest these heavily-processed acid ash foods, but it also has to try to shift your bloodstream towards alkalinity, and god forbid you have a kidney stone... Essentially, consuming a diet heavy in acid ash foods is a mess for the body, especially if you are an older individual, overweight, or already have health problems. Homeostasis is a state that your body goes to great length to reach and you can be a bro and help your body along a little bit.

Secret 7: A simple way of conceptualizing the Alkaline Diet is to think of it as a means that you can help your body achieve homeostasis by avoiding the typically acid ash foods of the Western diet and partaking in foods that shift the body away from acidosis.

The goal of this "secret" is merely to help you understand why the Alkaline Diet is more than a diet; it's a way of life. This diet is not merely a means for you to lose weight or achieve this goal or that. The Alkaline Diet is a way to help your body function normally, reduce your risk for various health problems down the line, increase your energy, and possibly even increase longevity.

Secret 8: The Alkaline Diet can be used to prevent osteoporosis in older individuals by reducing the acidosis of the blood thereby discouraging the body from metabolizing bone and encouraging bone deposition.

Good old Osteoporosis. Our old friend. The reason why we keep bringing it up is because this condition really represents one of the best examples of how the Alkaline Diet can change people's lives. It is also an example that illustrates that the Alkaline Diet isn't just another hokey diet, like some other diets that we will not name here. The Alkaline Diet is grounded in understanding the importance of pH in maintaining health and preventing the development of health conditions down the line. Though many people around the world will develop osteoporosis through no fault of their own, there are things you can do to help with your osteoporosis diagnosis or to at least delay it if you are getting close an age to this dreaded condition.

One of the ways that your body helps to maintain a homeostatic pH is by mobilizing alkaline substances from various parts of the body to raise the pH, and one of those locations is the bone. If you are already helping your body to be more alkaline, then you reduce the risk of your body mobilizing bone to fix the pH of the blood, and you also encourage the body to deposit bone rather than break down. This is a secret of the Alkaline Diet. This diet can actually push your body towards bone deposition rather than bone breakdown.

Secret 9: The Alkaline Diet can trigger weight loss as "alkaline ash" foods are often lower in calories than acid ash foods and frequently contain healthy antioxidants.

Although the primary goal of a dieter on the Alkaline Diet often is not weight loss, you can help push your body towards weight loss merely by consuming foods that are in the proper ratio of 80% from alkaline ash sources and 20% from acid ash sources. Again, what's great about this diet is that it comes with a host of unexpected advantages that most dieters were not thinking about when they decided on to embark on this diet.

You may have set sail on the Alkaline Diet thinking that you would prevent yourself from developing those painful kidney stones that you know run in the family, and, inadvertently, your skin has improved, your hair is thicker and shinier, you've lost some of that stubborn belly fat, and you might even have lengthened your life span. These are all things that you would have to be a fool to say "No" to.

Secret 10: Before you begin any diet, it is important to make a list of everything you hope to achieve while on your diet. This will both motivate you to continue your diet when times get a little rough, while also helping you to measure whether or not you are achieving the success you hoped for on your diet.

This is a secret that applies to any diet, but it is particularly important on this one as, for many of you, at least, your goal may not be purely weight loss. The good thing about having weight loss as a goal is that it should be relatively easy to tell if you are meeting this goal or not, right? You weight yourself one week in, two weeks in, three weeks in, etc. and you should be able to quantify if you are losing weight or not.

As many people on this diet will have other reasons for why they chose this one over others it will be important for you to keep track of whether or not you are meeting these goals. This is not only for practical reasons: what's the point of going to the farmer's market twice a week to get pomegranates and wheatgrass if you have no idea that the diet is working because you don't remember why you decided to go on it on the first place?

Don't get me wrong. It is perfectly all right to embark on a diet merely because you want to live a healthy lifestyle. Frankly, that is one of the better reasons to go on a diet. But if you did have specific reasons as to why you chose this diet, it would be important to keep track of those somehow, wouldn't it? That's a key secret to success on any diet.

CHAPTER 12

Tips to Ensure Alkaline Diet Success

Starting a new health journey is not easy. Things like poor eating habits are not easy to break. Because of this, you want to have a wealth of tips at your disposal to aid you in transitioning into your new diet and staying on track.

Making the Transition

Transitioning from your current diet to the alkaline diet is a lengthy process. Acknowledging this is important. If you try to make the drastic transition overnight, you are setting yourself up for failure. It is a good idea to get started about 30 days in advance. This gives you time to create goals, gradually change your eating habits and find a solid set of recipes for you to start learning how to make. If you make just a few changes a week for four weeks, by the time you reach week five, it will be much easier to completely stay on the alkaline diet.

Remember that with this diet, you are adding better things to your diet. Not only with nutrients and overall wholesomeness, but also with how much you can eat. Since the diet is largely plant-based, the foods you eat tend to contain far fewer calories. So, you can actually eat more frequently while cutting down on your calories. When you are meal planning, consider this so that you are eating enough each day.

Start experimenting with recipes during your 30-day transition phase. This way once you are fully doing the alkaline diet, you will have plenty of meals that you can enjoy and cook without issue. At this time, if you live with people and cook for them, you should also have them test your recipes. When the whole family transitions to the alkaline diet, it makes things much easier for you.

Start working on finding support. The internet is one of the best places for this. Head over to social media and start looking up groups specific to the alkaline diet. There is more than a dozen that is very active. Join several and determine which one or two you enjoy the most. Make sure to introduce yourself and just dive in feet first. You will meet fellow newbies that you can use as accountability buddies, as well as those well-versed in the diet that can answer your questions and help you make the right choices. Getting involved with these groups can also help to keep you motivated.

Make plans for mistakes. It is inevitable that you will slip up on occasion while you try to fully transition to the alkaline diet. If you make a plan for how to get back on track, these mistakes will not have a negative effect on your diet as a whole.

Stop thinking of it as a short-term diet. The alkaline diet is a lifestyle and something you can do for the rest of your life. Start thinking long-term and remember that you are changing your life for the better. This is not just a fix-it-quick method. You are doing something very positive for yourself.

Diet Tips that Work

The first step is to fully understand the alkaline diet. After reading this book, you will have accomplished this. Once you understand this diet, it makes it easier to follow because you will understand why you are making certain choices.

Create logical goals. Why do you want to use the alkaline diet? The answer to this question will make up your goals. For example, do you want to have more energy, reduce disease risk or lose weight? Write these down. When it comes to measurable goals, such as weight loss, break it down. For example, make a goal for every 10 pounds. As you hit the 10-pound milestone, this will help increase your motivation. Write your goals down and put them in a place you can easily see. For example, stick them in the fridge, so you see them all throughout the day. It is harder to disregard your goals when they are constantly in your face.

First and foremost, make sure to eat breakfast in the morning. This helps give your body the energy you need to get your day started. Secondly, most people are hungry in the morning. If you ignore this, you might find yourself tempted to make bad food choices mid-morning. A good breakfast also gives you about 15 minutes to just relax and think about the upcoming day. Use this time to prepare and savor your food.

The great thing about the alkaline diet is you can eat your main three meals, as well as one or two snacks, every day. Since you are eating relatively frequently and on a semi-regular schedule, it is much easier to avoid temptation. When you do not allow yourself to get hungry, it is easy to eat the right foods in the right portions.

Any successful diet is achieved by incorporating a wealth of vegetables and fruits into your diet. These are the backbone of the alkaline diet. These foods will provide you with all of your critical nutrients. They also give a lot of fiber, helping you to avoid premature hunger pangs.

Work on getting some exercise on a regular basis. If you have not gotten regular exercise in a while, see your doctor first. Once you get the go-ahead, start slow. For example, do three 10-minute sessions of exercise per day. You have to build up your endurance to do longer stints at a time. Make sure that the exercises you do are fun. For example, if you hate running, do not do it. If you love dancing, crank up some music and dance instead. Cardio is important, especially when you are trying to lose some weight. However, you also want to work on your flexibility and strength.

Water is critical for every diet. One benefit of the alkaline diet is that water is a staple and a lot of the common foods contain it. It is critical to stay hydrated and make sure you drink enough water every day. Not only does hydration help you feel more energetic, but it also prevents you from getting those dehydrated-related hunger pangs.

Make sure to read your food labels and scrutinize them. You want to know the nutrients especially so that you can ensure that you are properly fuelling your body. You also want to pay close attention to the ingredients. Some foods appear healthy and wholesome, but once you read the ingredients, you will find that certain foods are certainly not as healthy as the packaging makes them appear. Overall, foods that are not packaged because they're fresh are always the best choice.

Keep the foods to avoid out of your home. When 'bad' foods are present, and you see them frequently, the temptation will always be there, making it difficult for you. Remember the saying that when something is out of your sight, it is also out of your mind? This is very true, especially when it comes to foods. While you are preparing to start on the alkaline diet, go through your kitchen. Get rid of anything that does not fit within the guidelines of the alkaline diet.

Tips Specific to the Alkaline Diet

There are certain tips that are specific to the alkaline diet that can help you. Keep the following in mind as you transition into this diet:

- Ditch soda and drink water instead
- Start experimenting with sea vegetables as replacements for foods, such as egg noodles
- Use gourds and roots to start getting rid of the carbohydrates in your diet
- When drinking water, consider drinking the kind that's filtered
- Keep your animal proteins to a strict minimum (no more than one day at the very most)
- Avoid consuming alcohol since it contributes to acidity

- Start taking advantage of spices and herbs to flavor your food and add variation
- If you are planning to take supplements, speak with your healthcare provider first

Use as many of these tips as you can. When you put them into practice from day one, you will find that any challenges that you will face are much easier to overcome. It will also allow you to stay focused on your goals. The last tip to remember is that if you accidentally fall off track, do not beat yourself up over it. This happens to everyone. Simply correct your mistake immediately and get back on this diet.

CHAPTER 13

Beginner Mistakes

Now that we've covered health risks let's focus on some mistakes beginners usually make when they start with the alkaline way of nutrition. That way we can secure that you won't repeat these mistakes and that you will be on your way to achieving an alkaline lifestyle:

You Can't Reach Perfection Immediately

Whenever people start a diet, they have in mind that they need to strive for perfection. Whether a person is a young artist or an experienced engineer, they want to reach the alkaline goal immediately and be perfect from day one. The truth is – it's extremely hard to conduct any diet from the beginning entirely. Expecting too much is a sure way to failure. Starting the alkaline nutrition means that you should change your way of life and that is not something you can easily do. Furthermore, it just takes extreme effort and brings almost no fun and enjoyment.

Believe it or not, the fastest way to make a change in your life is to take it one step at a time. Remember, you are not only trying to implement new eating habits and foods, but you are also trying to give up the old ones. That requires a lot of work and persistence. That is why it is important to appreciate all the small steps you've made.

It's only natural that you will have an occasional setback. People often throw out the window everything that they have done up until that point once they make their first mistake. That's wrong!

The pressure is enormous – you need to fight the cravings, change your habits, fight your brain not to desire particular foods, and go through the everyday stress and work and/or in your private life. That is just too much to handle at once, so make sure to appreciate on everything you managed to do.

When it comes to alkaline diet, the important thing is to take care of some basics, such as staying hydrated and securing that your intake of green vegetables and minerals is at an adequate level.

It might be good advice to focus on implementing the things you like into your alkaline diet. Of course, these need to be the things that are in line with your new way of nutrition, but make sure to know what you like and keep your attention on that. If you need to eliminate a lot of highly acidic foods, try removing one at a time. For example, don't drink coffee anymore from this week, and start removing milk from the next week. When you are keeping it gradually, make sure to at least succeed in taking these smaller steps.

You Need to Think in Advance

If I learned something from people that successfully implemented a diet, it's that you always need to think in advance. I've personally faced a sudden crash in my way of nutrition due to a simple reason – I wasn't prepared.

A particular way of nutrition requires you to have certain meals. But when you've just come home from a stressful day at work, and you notice that there is nothing to eat, everything goes down the drain. If you add that it's rainy and cold outside and you don't feel like going to the store, ordering a pizza seems like a very good idea. And while you are waiting for it to arrive, grab that convenience food that has been in your cupboard for weeks.

Thinking in advance first means that you need to have enough of raw ingredients in your refrigerator to be able to whip up a meal whenever you need it. The other important thing in preparation is to know what you are going to cook. It's virtually impossible to invent a meal in a short amount of time, especially if you are looking for an alkaline-friendly dish that should also be tasteful.

My advice is to prepare a bunch or recipes that are easy, tasteful and alkaline-friendly. These meals should be dishes that you can always rely on. You should make sure to perform shopping regularly to secure that you have enough ingredients in your fridge.

A good idea is also to make a nutrition plan in advance. You don't just need to know what you are going to eat for lunch, but you also want to plan what you will eat for dinner tomorrow or two days for now. That's why it's important to make a menu of things you like and plan ahead. Whether you are on the alkaline or any other type of diet, it's crucial not to leave things to fate. Shopping and eating day-to-day is a big mistake – hunger, tiredness or any other reason will eventually cause you to disrupt your diet just because you weren't prepared. Instead, make sure that your refrigerator always has about a dozen of ingredients you can use to make different alkaline meals or snacks in a matter of minutes.

Proper Digestion

Proper digestion is essential for every diet, and it is crucial for the alkaline way of nutrition. After eating highly acidic foods for a while, they affect your digestive system by clogging it. Bacteria, yeast, candida, and mycotoxins all find their way to your gastrointestinal tract, meaning that your organism produces more waste and becomes more acidic. Irritable bowel syndrome is only one of the things that yeasts and bacteria can cause.

Aside from causing you problems, a much bigger worry is that your organism can only use a small portion of all those nutrients you have been consuming. Yeasts and other undigested matters coat the walls of your intestines and prevent nutrients from entering and your body to absorb them.

That is why it is incredibly important to cleanse your digestive system and allow it to function properly. That means that you will improve your nutrients absorption and, therefore, your diet results through no extra work!

Alkaline diet takes into account that your digestive system needs to be cleansed, but there are some additional steps you can take to speed up this process.

- Digestive foods – certain types of food can help you quickly detoxify your digestive system. These foods include avocado, greens, broccoli, celery, sweet potatoes, and chickpeas. When you feel like having a snack, go for grapefruit, which is mildly alkaline, and it contains pectin fiber, which is known as an excellent cleanser for the digestive system. On the other hand, make sure to avoid foods that are bad for you, such as trans-fats, processed foods, yeast, sugar, etc.

- Digestive supplements – you can use fiber supplements, such as psyllium husks. There are also other supplements that help your digestion, so make sure to check out for them in the local pharmacy or a drug store. The one thing you want to ensure is that they contain no sugar or artificial ingredients.

- Stay hydrated – once again, drinking enough fluids proves to be essential for your organism. Drinking enough water every day helps your digestive system and your entire body.

- Take your time with chewing – this is also known as premature swallowing, and it's caused by talking while eating and incomplete chewing. You see, the digestive system cannot digest big food chunks, so eating large pieces leads to digestive discomfort. The entire process of digestion actually starts in your mouth with chewing. On top of that, digestive enzymes that get released through chewing are essential for the further digestion process.

- Have enough time for a meal – if you are under stress or in a rush to head out, you can properly eat, and that also stresses your digestive system. When you are eating, you need to take your time. Every meal should be a way of relaxing. You should also make sure not to reach for your fork until you completely chew and swallow your current mouthful. There is no reason not to savor every bite and enjoy your meal.

Eat Regularly and Avoid Big Meals

Large meals impose a lot of stress on your digestive system. That is why it's important to eat on a regular basis and to eat smaller or moderate meals. Normal eating will also prevent you from feeling hungry quickly after a meal and keep you from having an unhealthy acidic snack.

The point of this section is to prove that the way of eating is equally important as what you eat. I'm sure that you felt bloated or suffered problems after you just induced a significant amount of food in a matter of minutes. The simple tips to help your digestive system will assist you in improving the results of your diet through no extra work.

Don't Be Afraid to Eat

When people start a new diet, they think that the goal is to eat as little as they can. They believe that small meals will help them get rid of those extra pounds. Believe it or not, this is wrong!

Yes, there is such thing as consuming too much food, but there is absolutely no reason to be restricted to small meals. Furthermore, when it comes to alkaline diet, the best way to clean your body of acids is to load it with nutrients. And what better way to secure you induced enough healthy ingredients than eating a lot?

Believe it or not, the worst thing you can do on the alkaline diet is to have a plain salad as your meal. You need to make sure that you induce enough of various foods to secure all the required nutrients to make your body slightly alkaline. As long as you follow the ratio of 80/20 for alkaline foods, you are good.

There is one thing to make sure on the alkaline diet – you shouldn't be hungry at any moment. Believe it or not, feeling hungry is an acidic state, so you need to make sure to avoid that from happening. If you are feeling hungry often, then you probably need to make some adjustments to your nutrition plan. Make sure not to miss any meals and vital nutrients that your body needs to work properly. Having three meals during the day is a must, and there is no reason not to throw in some healthy snacks, such as seeds or nuts, and even tomato or avocado.

CHAPTER 14:

Frequently Asked Questions

What is the Alkaline Diet?

The Alkaline Diet is a nutrition program that involves consuming certain foods in order to correct or prevent certain conditions associated with acidosis (low pH) of the blood or urine. The Alkaline Diet can also be used to achieve a general sense of health and wellness, for weight loss, and to achieve increased energy. The foods that one consumes on the Alkaline Diet help to shift the body away from acidosis because these foods are on the other end of the pH spectrum, they are alkaline (high pH).

Is the Alkaline Diet safe?

The Alkaline Diet is considered safe as it consists of foods that are generally regarded as healthier than other foods consumed in many diets. Many of your heavily processed foods and drinks are acid ash foods, which can easily be determined by reading food labels. Most processed or packaged foods contain acids or other compounds that are associated with making the body more acidotic. The Alkaline Diet does not involve consuming any strange or radical formulations, merely foods that can be easily obtained at a supermarket or farmer's market. As some people may be embarking on this diet for aid with a specific health condition, it is always a good idea to consult with your doctor or healthcare provider.

Is the Alkaline Diet the same as being a vegetarian or a vegan?

This is a good question. In reality, meats and fish (carnivorous foods) are all acid ash foods, so on an Alkaline Diet you would only be allowed to have about 20 percent of your food form sources like meat or fish, though you would be able to consume certain types of milk, though not other dairy products like cheese and eggs, which are considered acid ash foods. So, to answer your question, the Alkaline Ash diet can be a type of lacto-vegetarian diet, as the only animal product you would be able to consume in the alkaline ash percentage is certain types of milk, and some people choose to avoid meat, fish, and dairy altogether.

Can I drink milk on an Alkaline Diet?

Good question. Why is it a good question? Well, because there is not a consensus about this. Cow's milk is basic with a pH of about 7.33, but this is actually lower than the physiologic pH of humans of 7.4. Some nutritionists think it's okay, indeed, many of us were taught in school that milk is basic so it's a great way to counteract the activity of spicy foods! Though milk may be basic compared to many foods in the Western diet, technically, it is still lower than physiologic pH, therefore, again, you will have to decide whether you want to consume cow's milk. Goat's milk, however, is definitely part of the Alkaline Diet, as is Almond Milk.

What is the difference between acid ash and alkaline ash?

The terms "acid ash" and "alkaline ash" refer to the pH of the ash of foods after you combust them in a food combustion machine (that reduces them to ash). That's it. Acid ash foods have an acidic pH, that is pH below about 7.3, while alkaline ash foods have a basic or alkaline pH. The reason why this is important is because acid ash and alkaline ash foods have an effect on pH within the body; therefore, alkaline ash foods can be used to help correct states associated with acidosis in the body.

How does the Alkaline Diet help people with kidney stones?

The problem with kidney stones is that the blood and the urine, specifically, are acidotic, which can be easily measured with tests that measure pH, so the utility of the Alkaline Diet in this instance is in shifting your blood and urine toward a more alkaline pH, therefore preventing your kidneys from forming kidney stones. You may already know that the formation of kidney stones is associated with consumption of diets heavy in nitrogenous, acidic foods, like meat, for example. As you know, the Alkaline Diet does not include any meat and this would help you with kidney stones.

Does the Alkaline diet involve eating organic food?

There is not a clear cut relationship between the Alkaline Diet and whether a food is organic or not, as both alkaline ash foods and acid ash foods can be organic. Indeed, any alkaline ash foods may not be organic, so if consuming organic foods is important to you then you need to carefully read food labels (or shop at farmer's markets where they sell organic food).

Can the Alkaline Diet be incorporated with other diets?

We delve into this issue more deeply in a latter question, but it is definitely possible to incorporate the Alkaline Diet with other diets. This is easily accomplished as the Alkaline Diet focuses on what you are eating, not on how much or when. As you may already know, most diets fall under the Total Caloric Restriction category, meaning that they involve eating fewer calories as a mainstay of the diet. Other diets manipulate timing of when food is consumed (Intermittent Fasting) or play around with the ratio of one nutrient versus another (Ketogenic Diet). As this diet, again, is more about eating foods that are alkaline, it is not difficult to incorporate with other diets, you would just have to make sure that you are consuming foods that are in the Alkaline category.

Do I need to measure my pH while on the Alkaline Diet?

In this eBook we went into great detail explaining what pH was and why pH is an important part of the Alkaline Diet. As a quick review, the pH is essentially what tells us if our blood or urine is acidic, basic (alkaline) or neutral. For some people, their goal on this diet is to treat or prevent conditions associated with acidosis of the blood or urine. An Alkaline diet will shift the blood and urine away from acidosis by natural means through the consumption of alkaline ash foods. Some people may choose to measure the pH of their urine on this diet, especially if their concern is kidney stones, and there are several ways that one may measure the pH of the urine. In reality, it is not essential to measure pH of the blood or urine while on this diet.

Should I consult with a physician before I begin the Alkaline Diet?

Any person considering beginning a diet should consult their physician. This is particularly true in the case of the Alkaline Diet as many of you may be embarking on this diet with a specific goal of treating a health condition. The Alkaline Diet is healthy and the foods that are part of this diet are natural and organic, but when in doubt always ask your physician or health provider for guidance.

I occasionally go on fasts. Can I fast while on the Alkaline Diet?

Fasting is perfectly healthy and natural. Indeed, human beings have been fasting for many thousands of years, for both practical reasons and for religious or spiritual reasons. In fact, periods of fasting punctuated by shorter periods of eating is the normal way that our human ancestors would have eaten and lived in the earlier days of human history. They did not have fast food and soda, they did not have refrigerators, freezers, and processed foods to keep in the cupboards. They would not even have had cupboards. If they were hungry, these early humans would have to hunt and fish to satiate that hungry. Therefore, they would have had prolonged periods were they were not eating. It is the opinion of this book that fasts as perfectly healthy and can easily be incorporated into an Alkaline Diet. Naturally, any person with an underlying health problems that affect the absorption or metabolism of food, like diabetes mellitus, should consult a doctor before beginning any diet.

How will I know if my Alkaline Diet is working?

We talk about this later in some of the other questions, but the way that you will know if your diet is working will be a function of what your goals are on the diet. Many of you will begin this diet because you just want to feel healthier and you have heard that the Alkaline Diet is a fantastic way to steer your body in a healthier direction. Others of you will embark on the Alkaline Diet because you have a specific health issue and you would like to utilize this diet as part of the management of your health condition. If your goal is general health and wellness, you would measure your success on this diet by things like increased energy, less depression and anxiety, better skin tone resulting from less processed, acidic foods, and the like. If you are engaging in this diet for a specific health reason, then you would have to continue to utilize whatever means you use to keep track of your condition.

Can I expect weight loss while on the Alkaline Diet?

Many people on the Alkaline Diet experience weight loss, and this occurs for a number of reasons. One of the main reasons is that the Alkaline Diet steers you away from processed foods or other foods that screw with your metabolism (like heavy starches). Because of this, your body has to expend fewer calories to digest food, is less likely to store excess calories as fat (because you are not eating the acid ash foods that are associated with fat storage) and reaches homeostasis a little easier than it might otherwise.

I have an active fitness regimen. Will the Alkaline Diet interfere with my ability achieve my fitness goals? This is a common question for people starting any diet and it is a very important question to act. In general, the issue that people engaged actively in fitness will have on the Alkaline Diet is making the food requirements of this diet work for them in terms of their own macronutrient needs. Many of you active in the fitness world will have specific goals in terms of daily macronutrient consumption (fats, carbohydrates, and proteins) so you may have to make significant adjustments to your diet as many of the foods that you are used to eating will be acid ash foods. It is completely possible to meet your macronutrient goals while on an Alkaline Diet, though those of you with extremely high protein demands may have to make an adjustment. You can maintain a healthy protein intake while on the Alkaline Diet, but as this diet avoids the acid ash foods of most meats and dairy, then you would have to find other sources for your protein and possibly lower you protein quota a bit.

Is it difficult to stick to an Alkaline Diet?

It is not easy sticking to any diet. If it was, everyone would partake of diets and we all would achieve are dietary goals. In reality, many people who embark on diets fail and this is often a function of having unrealistic expectations on the diet or not being disciplined enough to stick to the diet.

Fortunately for many people, the Alkaline Diet includes many foods that people enjoy eating and the problem is not so much sticking to the diet, so to speak, but getting used to not eating foods that one may be used to eating, like sour or bitter fruits, meats, grains, and the like. In reality, it is no more difficult to stick to the diet than it is to stick to any other diet; indeed, it may be a bit easier as you are not restricting your caloric intake on this diet (unless you want to) as you would be on many other diets, like a Low Fat diet, or any other diet that involves Total Caloric Restriction.

What are the advantages of the Alkaline Diet compared to other diets?

This is not a simple question as ever dieter has their own individual reasons that determine why they choose to go on a diet in the first place, and why they might choose one particular diet over another. Many individuals that choose to go on a "diet" do so because their goal is weight loss or fat loss. In reality, a "diet" is nothing more than a specific eating regimen, therefore the goal of a diet does not have to be weight loss or fat loss.

If the goal of your diet is, in fact, weight loss the Alkaline Diet can help you achieve weight loss as the foods that are the staples of this diet are generally associated with less storage of excess calories in the form of fat, as well as improved metabolism and insulin resistance. These latter benefits are achieved on the Alkaline Diet as this diet does not include the grains and heavily processed foods that tend to steer us toward weight gain. Many other diets, however, can help you achieve your goal if your goal is weight loss. Diets that have been shown to be effective at weight loss include Intermittent Fasting, the Ketogenic Diet (of which Atkins is a type), and perhaps the most common diet, Total Caloric Restriction. Total Caloric Restriction is nothing more than the general term for a diet that is based around reducing your overall caloric intake in order to put you in a caloric deficit and encourage your body to burn fat for energy.

Though the Alkaline Diet can trigger weight loss, its advantages vis a vis other diets have more to do with its health benefits. The Alkaline Diet has been shown to prevent and also treat kidney stones, muscle wasting, osteoporosis, and various other diets associated with acidosis of the blood or urine. The Alkaline Diet helps the body maintain homeostasis, which is often difficult in the modern Western diet of processed foods and sodas that are acid ash foods that shift the blood toward acidosis and encourage harmful conditions like osteoporosis. Therefore, it is difficult to compare the Alkaline Diet to other diets as the goals of dieters in this particular diet are generally different from those in other diets.

What do I need to do to be successful on my Alkaline Diet?

A major component of being successful on a diet, including this one, is having a clear idea of your goals on this diet, as well as an idea of how you plan to accomplish those goals. As your plan as far as accomplishing your goals essentially involves following this diet to a "T", this e-book will do some of the work for you. If you plan to follow the Alkaline Diet closely, all you really need to do is eat the foods that fall under the alkaline ash category and avoid the acid ash foods. Another component of being successful on a diet is having a sense of how you are going to measure your goals. For example, if your goal on your diet is weight loss then naturally you need to make sure that you weight yourself on the first day of your diet and, say, once a week thereafter. As this is an

Alkaline Diet that we are talking about, many of you will have goals that involve a health condition perhaps or the prevention of a health condition. Therefore it might be more obvious to you if you are meeting your goals on this diet as the symptoms associated with your condition would diminish or disappear completely. And finally, people often feel healthier and more energetic on an Alkaline Diet as their body does not have to expend so much energy digesting food or keeping the body in homeostasis, so you should notice yourself feeling a little better on this diet. This is an indication of success, as well.

What is the approach of the medical community to the Alkaline Diet?

Good question. There is some controversy surrounding the Alkaline Diet in the medical community, primarily as there has been an assertion that some of the claims of the Alkaline Diet have not been verified. Although not every claim made by advocates of this diet has been backed by medical research, in reality, there is actually overlap between much of the ideas that are part of the Alkaline

Diet and suggestions made by doctors themselves. For example, doctors will normally advise people suffering from kidney stones to avoid certain foods and dietary practices, like consuming meals heavy with meats, and this is actually an important aspect of the Alkaline Diet as meats are considered acid ash foods. The long and short of it, there is not agreement between the medical and dietetic communities as far as this diet is concerned, although there is significant overlap between the suggestions made by both camps.

RECIPES

SALADS

Spaghetti Mushroom Salad

Ingredients:

- 300 g whole-wheat spaghetti
- 2 tablespoon sesame oil
- 2 minced garlic cloves
- 1 teaspoon minced ginger
- 2 teaspoon caraway seeds
- 60 g oyster mushrooms
- 100 g chopped kale leaves
- 2 tablespoons olive oil
- 2 chopped jalapeno pepper
- 2 tablespoons lemon juice
- Some chopped coriander
- 2 teaspoons salt
- **1 teaspoon pepper**

Directions:

1. Boil some water in a large vessel, throw in the spaghetti and cook for about 7-8 minutes. Drain the water and set aside.

2. In another sauce pan, take some olive oil, sauté the minced garlic, ginger, caraway seeds. This should take a few minutes.

3. Add the mushrooms, kale leaves, jalapeno chili, pepper, salt and stir fry for 3-4 minutes.

4. Once cooled down, transfer the mixture from the saucepan to a large bowl. Add the boiled noodles, sprinkle some lemon juice and toss well.

5. Garnish with some toasted sesame seeds and serve.

6. **Enjoy!**

Nutritional Information per Serving:

Calories: 362.5; Total Fat: 13.8g; Carbs: 47.1g; Protein: 16.2g

Noodle Salad with Broccoli

Ingredients:

- 150 g shitake or button mushrooms, chopped
- A handful of chopped and blanched kale leaves
- 160 g blanched broccoli florets
- 2 medium onion, sliced
- 4 tablespoons of olive oil
- 2 teaspoons pepper
- 1 teaspoon salt
- 100 g sprouts
- 2 teaspoons dark soy sauce
- 240 g soba noodles
- 1000 ml water to boil the noodles
- **Some chopped parsley for garnish**

Directions:

1. Take some water in a large sauce pan and bring it to a boil. Add half a teaspoon of olive oil so the noodles don't stick to each other.

2. Slide in the noodles and cook for about 3-4 minutes until they become slightly tender. Remember not to overcook the noodles. Drain the water. Set aside.

3. Take a salad bowl and mix the mushrooms along with kale leaves, broccoli florets, onion, noodles, pepper, salt, soy sauce and sprouts.

4. Drizzle some olive oil on top and toss.

5. Garnish with chopped parsley. Enjoy!

Nutritional Information per Serving:

Calories: 187.7; Total Fat: 11.1g; Carbs: 21.5g; Protein: 3.3g

Tomato Avocado Cucumber Salad

Ingredients:

- 2 avocados, peeled, pitted and sliced
- 4 big tomatoes
- 4 garlic cloves, minced
- 150 g arugula leaves
- 40 g cilantro
- 2 cucumbers, peeled and sliced
- 1 apple, peeled and sliced
- 200 g of basmati rice, cooked and cooled
- 60 g almonds
- A pinch of salt
- Juice of 2 lemons
- 120 ml coconut milk
- **1 teaspoon curry powder**

Directions:

1. Place all the salad ingredients in a bowl and stir well.
2. Mix lemon juice with coconut oil, Himalayan salt and curry powder.
3. Spread the salsa over the salad.
4. **Enjoy!**

Nutritional Information per Serving:
Calories: 90.2; Total Fat: 4.6g; Carbs: 10.7g; Protein: 3.3g

Spinach Bean Tomato Salad

Ingredients:

- 200 g chickpea, soaked overnight
- 160 g black beans, soaked overnight
- 4 cucumbers, peeled and chopped
- 2 medium onions, finely chopped
- 2 chopped tomatoes
- 2 chopped raw mangos
- 15 spinach leaves
- 2 teaspoons ground cumin
- 2 teaspoons raw mango powder
- 1 teaspoon salt
- 1 teaspoon cayenne pepper
- Some chopped cilantro
- **2x 1000 ml water to boil the beans and chickpeas**

Directions:

1. Boil the chickpeas and black beans in water. Drain and set aside.
2. Boil some additional water in another vessel and blanch the spinach for about 30 seconds. Drain the water.
3. In a large bowl, combine the chickpeas, blanched lettuce, cumin, onion, chopped raw mango, dry mango powder, pepper, tomato, salt and mix well.
4. Garnish with some chopped cilantro and serve.

5. Enjoy!

Nutritional Information per Serving:

Calories: 319.7; Total Fat: 22.8g; Carbs: 22.4g; Protein: 11.8g

Jalapeno Pomegranate Salad

Ingredients:

- 240 g chopped apples
- 300 g cucumber, peeled and sliced
- 300 g pomegranate seeds
- 2 Jalapeño Peppers
- 2 medium onions, peeled and chopped
- 25 raw almonds
- 2 minced garlic cloves
- 2 tablespoons lemon juice
- 1 teaspoon lemon zest
- A teaspoon of pepper powder
- 4 tablespoons raisins
- 16 lettuce leaves
- 1 teaspoon salt
- 2 tablespoons olive oil
- **A handful of wakame seaweed, previously soaked in water as per instructions**

Directions:

1. Combine all the ingredients in a big bowl, starting with all the veggies, then the fruits, wakame and spices.
2. Drizzle some olive oil on top and toss well. Add salt to taste.
3. **Serve immediately or refrigerate for 2 hours.**

Nutritional Information per Serving:

Calories: 83.5; Total Fat: 3.9g; Carbs: 12.1g; Protein: 1.9g

Detox Salad

Servings: 2

Prep time: 10 minutes

Ingredients

- 3 beets, peeled, roasted and diced
- 3 green onions, sliced
- 1 lime, juiced
- ¼ cup raisins
- 3 cups watercress
- 1 pear, diced
- 1 celery stalk, diced
- ½ avocado, diced
- ½ cup almonds, toasted and crushed

Dressing

- 1 garlic clove, minced
- ¼ teaspoon Himalayan salt
- 1 teaspoon coriander
- 1 teaspoon cumin
- ½ teaspoon cinnamon
- ½ teaspoon turmeric
- ½ teaspoon fresh ginger, grated
- 1 lemon, juiced
- 6 tablespoons of avocado oil

Directions

1. In a large bowl, combine beets, green onions, lime juice, raisins, watercress, pear, celery, avocado and almonds. Toss well to combine.

2. In a small bowl or jar, combine all the Dressing ingredients together. Whisk well to combine.

3. Pour Dressing over the beet and watercress mixture and toss well to coat.

4. Serve immediately.

Chopped Salad

Servings: 2
Prep time: 10 minutes

Ingredients

- ½ head romaine lettuce
- 1 cucumber, diced
- 1 tomato, diced
- ½ green bell pepper, diced
- ¼ cup green onions, diced
- ¼ cup black olives, chopped
- 2 tablespoons red onion, diced
- 2 tablespoons parsley, chopped

Dressing

- 1 tablespoon lemon juice
- 2 tablespoons apple cider vinegar
- 1 garlic clove, minced
- ¼ teaspoon Himalayan salt
- ⅛ teaspoon pepper
- ½ teaspoon dried oregano
- 1/3 cup olive oil

Directions

1. Make Dressing by whisking together all the Dressing ingredients together.

2. Place the lettuce, cucumber, tomato, bell pepper, green onions, olives, red onion and parsley in a large bowl. Drizzle with Dressing and toss to coat.

Tropical Tofu Salad

Servings: 2

Prep time: 10 minutes

Ingredients

- ½ mango, diced
- ½ cup pineapple, diced
- 1 carrot, shredded
- ½ red bell pepper, thinly sliced
- 7 ounces firm tofu, drained and diced
- ¼ cup cilantro, chopped
- 1 cup arugula
- ¼ cup sesame seeds, toasted
- 2 tablespoons green onions

Dressing

- 1 tablespoon white miso paste
- 2 teaspoons warm water
- 2 teaspoons coconut aminos
- 1 lime, juiced
- ¼ teaspoon cayenne pepper

Directions

1. Make Dressing by combining the Dressing ingredients in a small bowl and whisking well. If mixture is too thick or miso won't dissolve, add more warm water.

2. In a large bowl, combine the mango, pineapple, carrot, bell pepper, tofu, cilantro and arugula together.

3. Drizzle Dressing on top and toss to coat.

4. Sprinkle with sesame seeds and green onions.

Sweet Broccoli Quinoa Bowl

Servings: 2

Prep time: 10 minutes

Ingredients

- 5 tablespoons water
- 2 tablespoons tahini
- 1 teaspoon turmeric
- ½ teaspoon cinnamon
- ½ lemon, juiced
- 1 teaspoon maple syrup
- 1 head broccoli, florets finely chopped
- ¼ cup red grapes, halved
- ¼ cup almonds, chopped
- 1 cup quinoa, cooked
- 1 teaspoon Himalayan salt
- 1 teaspoon black pepper, crushed

Directions

1. In a small bowl, whisk together the water, tahini, turmeric, cinnamon, lemon juice and maple syrup until smooth.

2. In a large bowl, combine the broccoli, grapes, almonds and quinoa.

3. Pour tahini sauce over the broccoli and quinoa mixture and add salt and pepper.

4. Toss well to coat and serve.

Cooling Mint Salad

Servings: 2
Prep time: 10 minutes

Ingredients

- 2 cups spinach, chopped
- 2 cups radishes, thinly sliced
- 1 cucumber, diced
- 2 small red onions, cut in half and thinly sliced
- ¼ cup almonds, sliced

Mint & Citrus Dressing

- 1 tablespoon raw honey
- ¼ cup orange juice
- 1 tablespoon lemon juice
- 4 tablespoons olive oil
- 1 teaspoon Himalayan salt
- 1 teaspoon black pepper, crushed
- 1 cup fresh mint leaves, chopped

Directions

1. In a small bowl, whisk together the Mint & Citrus Dressing ingredients.
2. In a large bowl, combine the spinach, radishes, cucumber, red onion and almonds. Pour in Mint & Citrus Dressing and toss to coat.
3. Serve immediately.

Antioxidant Salad

Servings: 2

Prep time: 10 minutes

Ingredients

- 1 tablespoon coconut oil
- 1 teaspoon apple cider vinegar
- ¾ cup almonds, toasted
- 1 garlic clove, minced
- ½ cup quinoa, cooked
- 1/3 cup raisins
- ¼ cup blueberries
- 2 cups spinach, torn
- 1 handful of sesame seeds
- 1 teaspoon Himalayan salt

Directions

1. In a large bowl, toss together all ingredients and mix well.
2. Chill 5 minutes and serve.

Minted Quinoa Salad

Servings: 2

Prep time: 5 minutes

Ingredients

- ½ cup red quinoa, cooked
- ½ red bell pepper, diced
- ½ green bell pepper, diced
- ½ cucumber, diced
- 6 ounces chickpeas, cooked
- 1/3 cup mint leaves, thinly sliced
- ½ red onion, thinly sliced
- 2 tablespoons parsley, chopped
- 1 tablespoon pine nuts, toasted

Dressing

- 3 tablespoons olive oil
- 2 tablespoons lemon juice
- 1 tablespoon lemon zest
- ½ teaspoon Himalayan salt
- 1 teaspoon oregano

Directions

1. In a large bowl, combine quinoa, red and green bell peppers, cucumber, chickpeas, mint leaves and onion.

2. In a small bowl, whisk together the olive oil, lemon juice, lemon zest, salt and oregano.

3. Pour Dressing over the quinoa and vegetables.

4. Garnish with parsley and pine nuts before serving.

MAINS

Spaghetti Squash

Prep time: 10 minutes
Cooking time: 17 minutes
Servings: 6

Ingredients:

- 12 oz spaghetti squash
- 2 teaspoons coconut oil
- 5 oz green peas, steamed
- 1 oz shallot, diced
- 1 sweet pepper, chopped
- 1 oz walnuts, chopped
- ¼ teaspoon minced garlic
- ¼ cup quinoa, cooked

Directions:

1. Cut the spaghetti squash into the halves.
2. Place the coconut oil in the skillet and add butternut squash.
3. Roast it from each side for 5 minutes over the medium heat.
4. Meanwhile, mix up together the green peas, shallot, sweet pepper, walnuts, and minced garlic. Stir the mixture.
5. Then add quinoa and stir it.

6. Then transfer the roasted butternut squash in the baking tray.

7. Fill the butternut squash halves with the quinoa mixture and place in the oven.

8. Cook the meal for 12 minutes at 365 F.

9. Let the cooked meal chill little and serve!

Nutritional Information per Serving: Calories 115, fat 5.2, fiber 2.3, carbs 14.7, protein 4.1

Alkaline Hummus

Prep time: 10 minutes

Servings: 6

Ingredients:

- 1 cup organic chickpea, cooked
- 1 teaspoon tahini
- 1 lime, juiced
- ¼ teaspoon minced garlic
- ½ teaspoon ground coriander
- 1 oz olive oil

Directions:

1. Place the chickpeas in the blender.
2. Add tahini and lime juice.
3. Blend the mixture until smooth and soft.
4. Then add the minced garlic and ground coriander.
5. Add olive oil and blend the mixture until smooth.
6. Transfer the cooked hummus in the bowl and serve!

Nutritional Information per Serving: calories 166, fat 6.9, fiber 5.9, carbs 21.1, protein 6.6

Summer Light Salad

Prep time: 8 minutes

Cooking time: 3 minutes

Servings: 2

Ingredients:

- ½ avocado, cubed
- ¼ cup fresh cilantro, chopped
- ¾ cup fresh parsley, chopped
- 1 oz radish, sliced
- 1 zucchini, chopped
- ½ teaspoon salt
- ½ shallot, chopped
- 2 tablespoons lemon juice
- 1 tablespoon olive oil
- ¼ teaspoon flax seeds

Directions:

1. Steam the zucchini for 2-3 minutes and put in the salad bowl.
2. Add chopped cilantro and parsley.
3. Then add radish and stir it.
4. After this, sprinkle the salad with the salt, shallot, lemon juice, and olive oil.
5. Stir it.
6. Add avocado and flax seeds. Shake it gently and serve!

Nutritional Information per Serving: calories 194, fat 17.4, fiber 5.6, carbs 10, protein 3.1

Alkaline Skewers

Prep time: 10 minutes
Cooking time: 10 minutes
Servings: 2

Ingredients:

- 1 red onion
- 1 zucchini
- 1 cup cherry tomatoes
- 2 garlic cloves
- 1 tablespoon olive oil
- ½ teaspoon ground coriander
- ¼ teaspoon salt
- 1 sweet pepper

Directions:

1. Remove the seeds from the sweet pepper and cut into the squares.
2. Then cut the zucchini into the big cubes.
3. Chop the onion roughly.
4. Skewer all the vegetables onto the skewers.
5. Then sprinkle the vegetables with the salt and ground coriander.
6. Sprinkle the skewers with the olive oil and place on the baking tray.
7. Cook the skewers for 10 minutes at 365 F.
8. Then serve the cooked meal immediately!

Nutritional Information per Serving: calories 137, fat 7.6, fiber 4.2, carbs 17.4, protein 3.4

Radish Bowl

Prep time: 5 minutes

Servings: 4

Ingredients:

- 2 cups radishes, sliced
- ¼ cup Greek-style yogurt
- ¼ teaspoon salt
- ¼ cup fresh parsley, chopped
- 1 teaspoon ground black pepper

Directions:

1. Place the sliced radishes in the bowl and sprinkle with the salt and ground black pepper.
2. Add chopped parsley and stir.
3. After this, add yogurt and stir it well.
4. Serve the cooked meal immediately!

Nutritional Information per Serving: calories 26, fat 0.5, fiber 1.2, carbs 4.6, protein 1.3

Lentil Pate

Prep time: 15 minutes

Cooking time: 20 minutes

Servings: 6

Ingredients:

- 1 ½ cup lentils, soaked
- 3 cups water
- 5 oz carrot, grated
- ½ teaspoon salt
- 1 white onion, diced
- 6 oz sweet pepper, chopped
- 2 oz tomato, chopped
- 1 teaspoon ground coriander
- ½ teaspoon ground ginger
- ½ teaspoon ground black pepper
- ¼ teaspoon smoked paprika
- 1 tablespoon olive oil
- 3 tablespoons lime juice

Directions:

1. Put the lentils, carrot, and water in the big pan and simmer for 15 minutes with the closed lid.
2. Meanwhile, pour the olive oil into the pan and preheat.
3. Add sweet pepper, tomato, and onion. Saute it for 4 minutes.

4. After this, transfer the vegetables to the blender.
5. Add the cooked lentils mixture and all the ingredients from the list above.
6. Blend the mixture until smooth and chill it well.
7. Serve the pate warm!

Nutritional Information per Serving: calories 253, fat 3.2, fiber 17.5, carbs 44.4, protein 14.2

Marinated Kale Salad

Prep time: 15 minutes

Cooking time: 15 minutes

Servings: 8

Ingredients:

- 1 sweet potato, peeled, cubed
- 1 white onion, roughly chopped
- 1 tablespoon coconut oil
- 1 tablespoon olive oil
- 1 teaspoon ground black pepper
- ½ teaspoon salt
- 7 oz beet, cubed
- 3 tablespoons lemon juice
- 2 cups kale

Directions:

1. Cover the baking tray with the parchment and place the sweet potato, onion, and beet there.
2. Sprinkle the vegetables with the salt and coconut oil and cook in the oven at 365 F for 15 minutes.
3. Meanwhile, chop the kale roughly and sprinkle with the ground black pepper, olive oil, and lemon juice.
4. Stir it well and let to marinate for 15 minutes.
5. When the vegetables are baked chill them till they are warm and place on the serving plates.
6. Add the marinated kale and serve immediately!

Nutritional Information per Serving: calories 69, fat 3.6, fiber 1.6, carbs 8.7, protein 1.4

Lentils Stew

Prep time: 10 minutes
Cooking time: 25 minutes
Servings: 4

Ingredients:

- 1 cup lentils, cooked
- 1 carrot, grated
- 1 white onion, diced
- 1 teaspoon salt
- 1 tablespoon coconut oil
- 1 tablespoon flax seeds
- 2 tomatoes, chopped
- 1 teaspoon ground black pepper
- 2 cups water

Directions:

1. Place the lentils and water in the saucepan.
2. Add ground black pepper and salt.
3. Close the lid and cook the lentils for 5 minutes over the medium heat.
4. Meanwhile, put the coconut oil in the pan and preheat it.
5. Add the diced onion and grated carrot.
6. Saute the vegetables for 5 minutes and add tomatoes. Stir the vegetables and cook them for 5 minutes more.

7. After this, add the vegetables to the lentils and stir well.

8. Close the lid and saute the stew for 10 minutes more over the low heat.

9. Then add the flax seeds and stir well.

10. Serve!

Nutritional Information per Serving: calories 238, fat 4.6, fiber 17, carbs 36.1, protein 13.7

Alkaline Minestrone

Prep time: 10 minutes

Cooking time: 25 minutes

Servings: 2

Ingredients:

- 2 teaspoons olive oil
- 1 leek, chopped
- 1 carrot, chopped
- 1 oz celery stalk, chopped
- ¼ cup finger potatoes, halved
- 4 oz frozen peas
- 1 oz fresh parsley, chopped
- 1 teaspoon salt
- ½ teaspoon ground black pepper
- 2 cups water

Directions:

1. Pour olive oil in the soup pan and add chopped leek and carrot.
2. Roast the vegetables for 3 minutes over the medium heat.
3. After this, add a celery stalk and finger potatoes. Stir the vegetables and cook for 2 minutes more.
4. Then add frozen peas, salt, ground black pepper, and water.
5. Stir it and close the lid.

6. Cook the soup over the medium heat for 10 minutes.

7. Then add the fresh parsley and cook the minestrone for 5 minutes more.

8. Chill the cooked minestrone until warm and serve!

Nutritional Information per Serving: calories 133, fat 5.1, fiber 5.5, carbs 19.1, protein 4.4

Mint Soup

Prep time: 15 minutes

Servings: 4

Ingredients:

- 4 cups water
- ½ teaspoon salt
- 1 teaspoon smoked paprika
- 2 avocados, peeled, pitted
- 1 cucumber, chopped
- 3 oz fresh mint leaves
- 1 oz lemon juice
- 1 teaspoon minced garlic

Directions:

1. Chop the avocados roughly and place in the blender.
2. Add smoked paprika, cucumber, mint leaves, and lemon juice.
3. Then add the minced garlic and blend the vegetables on the maximum speed for 1 minute.
4. Add water and blend the soup for 30 seconds more.
5. Ladle the cooked soup into the bowls and serve immediately!

Nutritional Information per Serving: calories 230, fat 20, fiber 8.8, carbs 13.8, protein 3.3

Carrot Soup

Prep time: 10 minutes

Cooking time: 25 minutes

Servings: 4

Ingredients:

- 3 teaspoons olive oil
- 5 oz onion, diced
- 4 cups vegetable broth
- 4 carrots, chopped
- 1 oz grated ginger
- ½ teaspoon salt
- 2 tablespoons Greek Style yogurt

Directions:

1. Pour the olive oil into the saucepan and add the diced onion.
2. Saute the onion until it is soft.
3. Then add the chopped carrot and grated ginger.
4. Stir it and saute for 5 minutes.
5. Add salt and vegetable broth.
6. Close the lid and cook the soup for 15 minutes over the medium heat.
7. Then add yogurt and blend the soup with the help of the hand blender until smooth.
8. Simmer the soup for 2 minutes more.
9. Enjoy!

Nutritional Information per Serving: calories 141, fat 5.5, fiber 3.2, carbs 16.5, protein 6.9

Ginger Snap Peas

Prep time: 10 minutes

Cooking time: 5 minutes

Servings: 2

Ingredients:

- 1 cup sugar snap peas
- 2 teaspoons olive oil
- ¼ teaspoon grated fresh ginger
- 1 teaspoon maple syrup
- 1 scallion, chopped
- 1 tablespoon orange juice
- 1 cup water
- ¼ teaspoon sea salt

Directions:

1. Pour water into the saucepan and bring it to boil.
2. Then add the sugar snap peas and boil them for 10 seconds or until they start to be green.
3. Transfer the cooked peas in the colander and chill in the ice water.
4. Then pour the olive oil in the skillet.
5. Add ginger and maple syrup.
6. Then add chopped scallion and orange juice.
7. Add sea salt and saute the liquid for 30 seconds.
8. Then add the peas and stir them well.
9. Cook the snap peas for 2 minutes more.

10. **10.** Enjoy!

Nutritional Information per Serving: calories 69, fat 4.8, fiber 1.1, carbs 6.1, protein 1.1

Tabouli

Prep time: 20 minutes
Cooking time: 1 hour
Servings: 6

Ingredients:

- 1-pound cauliflower head
- 1 cup fresh parsley, chopped
- 1 cup tomatoes, chopped
- 1 scallion, chopped
- 1 cucumber, chopped
- 3 tablespoons olive oil
- 2 tablespoons lime juice
- 1 teaspoon fresh mint
- ½ teaspoon salt
- 1 teaspoon ground black pepper

Directions:

1. Chop the cauliflower and place in the blender.
2. Blend the vegetable until you get the shape of tiny pieces (rice).
3. Then transfer the cauliflower rice in the big bowl.
4. Add chopped parsley, tomatoes, scallion, cucumber, and fresh mint. Stir it.
5. Sprinkle the mixture with the olive oil, lime juice, salt, and ground black pepper.
6. Stir the tabouli well and serve. Enjoy!

Nutritional Information per Serving: calories 103, fat 7.2, fiber 1.2, carbs 5.3, protein 1.1

Roasted Soup

Prep time: 10 minutes

Cooking time: 20 minutes

Servings: 5

Ingredients:

- 1 cup tomatoes, chopped
- 2 sweet peppers, chopped
- ½ cup onion, diced
- 1 tablespoon olive oil
- ½ teaspoon salt
- ½ teaspoon chili flakes
- ½ cup fresh parsley, chopped
- 1 teaspoon ground black pepper
- 5 cups water

Directions:

1. Pour the olive oil into the saucepan and add diced onion.
2. Saute the onion for 3 minutes over the medium heat.
3. Then add salt, chili flakes, ground black pepper, and chopped peppers.
4. Saute the vegetables for 2 minutes more.
5. After this, add tomatoes and water.
6. Close the lid and cook the soup for 10 minutes more over the medium heat.

7. Add the chopped parsley and cook it for 2 minutes more.

8. Chill the soup till the room temperature and ladle in the bowls.

9. Enjoy!

Nutritional Information per Serving: calories 54, fat 3.1, fiber 1.6, carbs 6.7, protein 1.2

DRINKS

Alkaline Veggie Juice

Servings: 2
Prep time: 5 minutes

Ingredients

- 2 carrots
- 1 cucumber
- ¼ head green cabbage
- 1 cup kale
- ½ lemon
- ½ cup parsley
- 1 inch piece ginger
- 1 inch piece turmeric

Directions

1. Place all ingredients in a juicer and serve immediately.

Coconut Lime Smoothie

Servings: 1
Prep time: 5 minutes

Ingredients

- 4 ounces fresh coconut meat
- ½ cup coconut water
- ½ cup coconut milk
- 1 tablespoon coconut oil
- 1 lime, peeled
- 1 banana, frozen
- 3 - 4 ice cubes
- ½ teaspoon lime zest

Directions

1. Place all ingredients except the lime zest in a blender and blend on high until fully combined.
2. Garnish with lime zest and serve.

Berry Blast Smoothie

Servings: 1

Prep time: 5 minutes

Ingredients

- 1 cup spinach
- ¼ cup blueberries
- ¼ cup raspberries
- 1 tablespoon raw cashew butter
- 1 tablespoon ground flaxseed
- 1 tablespoon coconut oil
- 1 cup almond milk
- 1 tablespoon chia seeds
- 1 tablespoon hemp hearts

Directions

1. Place all ingredients except the chia seeds and hemp hearts in a blender and combine.
2. Stir in chia and hemp hearts and serve.

Minty Morning Shake

Servings: 2

Prep time: 5 minutes

Ingredients

- ¾ cup unsweetened coconut milk
- ¼ cup canned coconut milk
- 1 cup fresh spinach
- ½ avocado
- ½ cup fresh mint leaves
- 2 bananas, frozen
- 2 dates, pitted
- 1 teaspoon vanilla extract
- ¼ teaspoon Himalayan salt
- ¼ teaspoon peppermint extract
- 6 - 8 ice cubes
- 1 teaspoon cacao nibs
- 2 fresh mint leaves

Directions

1. Place all ingredients except the cacao nibs and 2 fresh mint leaves in a blender until smooth.
2. Garnish with cacao nibs and mint leaves before serving.

Green Tea & Fruit Smoothie

Servings: 2

Prep time: 5 minutes

Ingredients

- 2 ripe mangoes, peeled and chopped
- ½ cup raspberries
- ¼ cup pineapple, diced
- 1 ripe frozen banana, peeled
- 1 cup unsweetened almond milk
- 1 lime, juiced
- 2 teaspoons matcha green tea powder
- 3 - 4 ice cubes

Directions

1. In a blender combine all ingredients until smooth and serve.

Apple Pie Smoothie

Servings: 2

Prep time: 5 minutes

Ingredients

- 1 red apple, cored and chopped
- ½ frozen banana
- 1 ½ cups unsweetened almond milk
- 3 dates, pitted, soaked for 15 minutes and drained
- 1 teaspoon cinnamon
- ½ teaspoon nutmeg
- ½ teaspoon vanilla extract
- ¼ teaspoon Himalayan salt

Directions

1. In a blender combine all ingredients until smooth and serve.

Morning Alkaline Lemon Water

Servings: 1

Prep time: 2 minutes

Ingredients

- 8 ounces of alkaline water, either lukewarm or slightly warmed (not boiling)
- ½ lemon, juiced

Directions

1. In a cup mix together the water and lemon juice.
2. Serve immediately either first thing upon waking (before consuming breakfast or other beverages) or before a meal.

Detox Juice

Servings: 1
Prep time: 5 minutes

Ingredients

- 2 small beets, peeled
- 1 carrot, peeled
- 1 small apple
- 1 lemon, peeled and seeds removed
- 1 ½ inch piece of ginger

Directions

1. Place all ingredients in your juicer and serve immediately.

Fruity Summer Lemonade

Servings: 2

Prep time: 2 minutes

Ingredients

- 3 lemons
- 1 apple
- 1 ½ cups water
- 1 cup fresh strawberries, washed and hulled
- 1 cup watermelon, cubed
- ½ cup mint
- 1 teaspoon raw honey
- 5-6 ice cubes

Directions

1. Juice lemons in a juicer and set aside the juice.
2. Juice apples in a juicer and combine juice with lemon juice in a blender.
3. Add water, strawberries, watermelon, mint, honey and ice cubes to the blender and blend until smooth.
4. Serve immediately.

All Day Detox Water

Servings: 2

Prep time: 2 minutes

Ingredients

- 16 ounces water
- 6 lemon slices
- 10 cucumber slices
- ¼ teaspoon Himalayan salt
- 5 - 6 ice cubes (optional)

Directions

1. In a small pitcher, combine water, lemon, cucumber, salt and ice cubes (if using).

Watermelon Mint Water

Servings: 2

Prep time: 2 minutes

Ingredients

- 16 ounces water
- ½ cup watermelon, cubed
- 8 mint leaves, torn
- ¼ teaspoon Himalayan salt
- 5 - 6 ice cubes (optional)

Directions

1. In a small bowl, using the back end of a spoon, muddle together the watermelon, mint and salt.

2. Add watermelon mint mixture to a pitcher and fill with water and ice cubes (if using).

Glow Juice

Servings: 2

Prep time: 5 minutes

Ingredients

- 2 green apples
- 1 cup collard greens, chopped
- 1 cup parsley
- ½ large cucumber
- 1 inch piece of ginger

Directions

1. Place all ingredients in juicer. Serve juice immediately.

DESSERTS

Apple Tart

Prep time: 5 minutes
Cooking time: 15 minutes
Servings: 6

Ingredients:

- ½ cup pecans
- ¼ cup almonds
- 2 oz dates
- ¾ teaspoon nutmeg
- 1 tablespoon coconut oil
- 1 teaspoon water
- ½ teaspoon vanilla extract
- 2 tablespoons lemon juice
- 2 sour apples
- 1 tablespoon agave syrup
- 1 teaspoon ground cinnamon
- 1 tablespoon coconut flakes

Directions:

1. Put the pecans, almonds, dates, and nutmeg in the blender.
2. Add coconut oil and water.

3. After this, add vanilla extract and blend the mixture until smooth.

4. Transfer the mixture in the tart mold and press it well to make the pie crust.

5. Then slice the apples and sprinkle them with the lemon juice.

6. Then place the apples in the pie crust and sprinkle with the agave syrup, ground cinnamon, and coconut flakes.

7. Chill the tart in the fridge for 5 minutes and serve!

Nutritional Information per Serving: calories 207, fat 13.2, fiber 4.7, carbs 23.4, protein 2.6

Buckwheat Smoothie

Prep time: 5 minutes

Servings: 4

Ingredients:

- 1 cup almond milk
- 1 cup water
- ½ cup buckwheat, soaked
- 1 cup strawberries
- ¼ cup agave syrup
- 1 tablespoon flax seeds

Directions:

1. Place the almond milk, water, buckwheat, strawberries, and agave syrup in the food processor.
2. Blend the mixture until smooth.
3. After this, pour the smoothie into the glasses and sprinkle with the flax seeds.
4. Enjoy!

Nutritional Information per Serving: calories 295, fat 15.7, fiber 4.7, carbs 38.4, protein 4.8

Banana Ice Cream

Prep time: 10 minutes

Cooking time: 2 hours

Servings: 1

Ingredients:

- 1 banana
- 2 dates
- 1 oz coconut meat, chopped
- ¼ teaspoon ground cinnamon

Directions:

1. Peel the banana and chop it.
2. Put the chopped banana in the blender.
3. Add dates and coconut meat.
4. Add ground cinnamon and blend the mixture until smooth.
5. Then put the mixture in the bowl or ice cream molds and place in the freezer.
6. Freeze the ice cream for 2 hours.
7. Enjoy!

Nutritional Information per Serving: calories 254, fat 9.9, fiber 7.3, carbs 44.2, protein 2.7

Rhubarb Pudding

Prep time: 10 minutes

Cooking time: 15 minutes

Servings: 4

Ingredients:

- 6 oz rhubarb
- 1 cup raspberries
- 1 cup fresh apple juice
- ½ teaspoon vanilla extract
- ¼ cup agave syrup
- 6 oz beet, juiced

Directions:

1. Preheat the oven to 365 F.
2. Chop the rhubarb and place in the baking tray.
3. Add the fresh apple juice and transfer to the oven.
4. Cook the rhubarb for 15 minutes.
5. Meanwhile, place the raspberry in the blender.
6. Add vanilla extract, agave syrup, and beet juice.
7. Blend the mixture until smooth.
8. When the rhubarb is cooked – add it in the blender and blend for 30 seconds more.
9. Serve the rhubarb pudding immediately!

Nutritional Information per Serving: calories 136, fat 0.5, fiber 3.8, carbs 33.5, protein 1.5

Strawberry Crumble

Prep time: 15 minutes

Servings: 2

Ingredients:

- 1 cup strawberries
- 2 tablespoons agave syrup
- ½ teaspoon vanilla extract
- 1 tablespoon lemon juice
- ½ cup almonds
- 4 dates

Directions:

1. Place the lemon juice, almonds, and dates in the blender.
2. Blend well.
3. Then place the almond mixture in the serving glasses.
4. Put the strawberries and agave syrup in the blender. Add vanilla extract and blend the mixture until smooth.
5. Pour the strawberry mixture over the almond mixture.
6. Stir the crumble gently.
7. Enjoy!

Nutritional Information per Serving: calories 276, fat 12.2, fiber 5.8, carbs 40.1, protein 6

Avocado Ice Cream

Prep time: 10 minutes
Cooking time: 2 hours
Servings: 4

Ingredients:

- 1 avocado, peeled, pitted
- 1 cup cherries, pitted, chopped
- 2 oz cashews, soaked
- 3 tablespoons water
- ½ teaspoon vanilla extract
- 4 oz dates, chopped
- 8 oz coconut milk

Directions:

1. Blend together the avocado, cherries, cashews, water, vanilla extract, and chopped dates.
2. When the mixture is smooth – add the coconut milk and blend the mixture for 1 minute more.
3. Pour the mixture into the ice cream maker and cook the ice cream according to the directions of the manufacturer.
4. Transfer the cooked ice cream in the ice cream molds and freeze for 2 hours.
5. Enjoy!

Nutritional Information per Serving: calories 438, fat 30, fiber 7.5, carbs 43.8, protein 5.3

Berry Steamer

Prep time: 5 minutes

Cooking time: 5 minutes

Servings: 3

Ingredients:

- 2 cups almond milk
- 1 cup strawberries, chopped
- 1 tablespoon coconut flakes
- ½ teaspoon vanilla extract

Directions:

1. Put the strawberries in the blender and blend until smooth.
2. After this, pour the almond milk into the saucepan and bring to boil.
3. Immediately remove the almond milk from the heat and transfer in the blender.
4. Add coconut flakes and vanilla extract.
5. Blend the strawberry mixture until smooth and you get the light foam.
6. Transfer the steamer in the bowls and enjoy!

Nutritional Information per Serving: calories 391, fat 38.8, fiber 4.6, carbs 12.9, protein 4

Pie-To Go

Prep time: 15 minutes

Servings: 2

Ingredients:

- 1/3 cup buckwheat, soaked
- ¼ teaspoon vanilla extract
- ¼ teaspoon ground cinnamon
- ¼ teaspoon ground ginger
- 1 tablespoon orange juice
- ½ teaspoon liquid stevia
- 2 oz cranberries
- 1 oz dates, chopped
- 2 tablespoons maple syrup
- 1 teaspoon lemon juice

Directions:

1. Mix up together the buckwheat, vanilla extract, ground cinnamon, and orange juice. Stir the mixture.
2. Place ½ part of the buckwheat mixture in the mason jars.
3. After this, place the cranberries, liquid stevia, ground ginger, dates, maple syrup, and lemon juice in the blender.
4. Blend until smooth.
5. Then pour the mixture into the mason jars.

6. Top the meal with the remaining buckwheat mixture and serve!

Nutritional Information per Serving: calories 212, fat 1.1, fiber 5.2, carbs 48.2, protein 4.2

Date Pudding

Prep time: 10 minutes

Servings: 4

Ingredients:

- 3 oz dates, chopped
- 1 avocado, peeled, pitted
- 1 teaspoon agave syrup
- ½ teaspoon ground cinnamon
- ½ cup blueberries
- ½ cup almond milk
- 1 teaspoon chia seeds
- 1 teaspoon flax seeds

Directions:

1. Chop the avocado and place it in the blender.
2. Add dates, agave syrup, ground cinnamon, and blueberries.
3. Then add almond milk and blend the mixture until smooth.
4. Transfer the pudding in the serving dishes and sprinkle with chia seeds and flax seeds.
5. Enjoy!

Nutritional Information per Serving: calories 260, fat 17.8, fiber 7.1, carbs 27.1, 2.7

Punch

Prep time: 20 minutes

Servings: 6

Ingredients:

- 3 lemons
- 3 cups strawberries
- 2 apples, chopped
- 2 cups water
- ¼ cup agave syrup

Directions:

1. Cut the lemons into halves and squeeze the juice with the help of the juicer.
2. Then place the strawberries in the blender and blend well.
3. Mix up together the blended strawberries and lemon juice. Add agave syrup and stir it.
4. Juice the apples and add the liquid to the lemon mixture. Add water.
5. Stir it well and serve!

Nutritional Information per Serving: calories 112, fat 0.4, fiber 4.1, carbs 29.6, protein 1

Tropicana Monkey

Prep time: 10 minutes

Servings: 4

Ingredients:

- 4 bananas, frozen
- 2 oz cocoa powder
- ¼ tablespoon cocoa nibs
- 10 oz almond milk
- 4 teaspoons chia seeds
- 1 tablespoon coconut oil

Directions:

1. Put the frozen bananas in the blender and add cocoa powder, cocoa nibs, and almond milk.
2. Then add coconut oil and blend well.
3. When the mixture is smooth – transfer it to the serving jars.
4. Sprinkle the meal with the chia seeds.
5. Enjoy!

Nutritional Information per Serving: calories 366, fat 25, fiber 11.4, carbs 41.8 protein 6.7

Parfait

Prep time: 10 minutes

Cooking time: 15 minutes

Servings: 2

Ingredients:

- 1 oz cashews, soaked
- ¼ cup almond milk
- ½ cup blueberries
- 2 tablespoons rolled oats
- 1 tablespoon chia seeds

Directions:

1. Blend together the cashews and almond milk until smooth.
2. Then place 1 tablespoon of the rolled oats in the mason jar.
3. Add the small amount of the cashew smooth mixture and blueberries.
4. After this, add rolled oats and all the remaining blueberries.
5. Add the remaining cashew mixture and sprinkle with the chia seeds.
6. Leave the parfait for 15 minutes in the fridge.
7. Enjoy!

Nutritional Information per Serving: calories 225, fat 16.4, fiber 5.5, carbs 18.5, protein 5.3

Chocolate Fro-Yo

Prep time: 15 minutes

Servings: 1

Ingredients:

- 1 banana, chopped, frozen
- ½ teaspoon cocoa powder
- 1 teaspoon almond butter
- 2 oz almond milk
- ¼ teaspoon hemp seeds

Directions:

1. Mix up together the frozen banana and cocoa powder in the blender.
2. Add almond butter and blend until smooth.
3. Transfer the mixture to the serving dish and add almond milk.
4. Stir well until homogenous.
5. Then sprinkle the meal with the hemp seeds and serve!

Nutritional Information per Serving: calories 339, fat 23.3, fiber 6.2, carbs 33.6, protein 6.4

CONCLUSION

Take baby steps instead of trying to launch full-force into this diet. Since this diet is meant to be more of a long-term lifestyle change, the last thing you want to do is burn yourself out too soon. It may be as simple as trying to start by eliminating excess sugar from your diet, and introduce more vegetables. From there, you can continue to eliminate problem acid foods and continue augmenting with vegetables and alkaline substitutes.

As you progress, you'll see very real results in your well-being and the way you feel, and it will be just the motivation you need to forge ahead. The most important thing you can do at that point is to make it your own. Many people make the mistake of trying to follow diet books and guides to a T.

The problem with this approach is that everyone's body is different and everyone's eating habits, motivations, and patterns are slightly unique. If you can make the alkaline diet your own, and approach it with your own unique style, you'll find it much easier to stay committed.

THANKS FOR READING!

What did you think of, The Alkaline Diet Made Easy: Reclaim Your Health, Lose Weight & Heal Naturally

I know you could have picked any number of books to read, but you picked this book and for that I am extremely grateful.

I hope that it added at value and quality to your everyday life. If so, it would be really nice if you could share this book with your friends and family by posting to Facebook and Twitter.

If you enjoyed this book and found some benefit in reading this, I'd like to hear from you and hope that you could take some time to post a review. Your feedback and support will help this author to greatly improve his writing craft for future projects and make this book even better.

I want you, the reader, to know that your review is very important and so, if you'd like to leave a review, all you have to do is click here and away you go. I wish you all the best in your future success!

Thank you and good luck!

Madison Fuller

Claim This Now

Autoimmune Healing Transform Your Health, Reduce Inflammation, Heal the Immune System and Start Living Healthy

Do you have an overall sense of not feeling your best, but it has been going on so long that it's actually normal to you?

If you answered yes to any of these question, you may have an autoimmune disease.

Autoimmune diseases are one of the ten leading causes of death for women in all age groups and they affect nearly 25 million Americans.

In fact millions of people worldwide suffer from autoimmunity whether they know it or not.

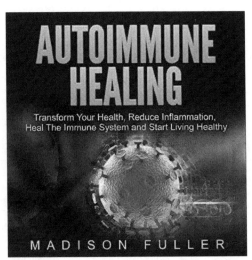

Want More?

Sign up to get the exclusive Madison Fuller e-newsletter, sent out a few times a week:

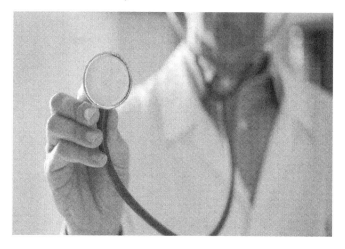

https://www.subscribepage.com/autoimmune

Made in the USA
Columbia, SC
02 February 2022

55251508R00119